Working More Creatively with Groups

In this classic text Jarlath Benson presents the basic knowledge required to set up and work with a group. He looks at how to plan and lead a group successfully and how to intervene skilfully. As well as covering the different stages in the life of a group, the book emphasizes the various levels of group experience and gives suggestions for working more creatively with them.

For this new edition the author has added two new chapters reflecting how his own thinking and practice have developed since the book was first published. In the first he presents a new model for understanding human behaviour which emphasizes particular contexts for work in groups: the psychophysical, the psychological, the psychosocial/cultural/political and the psychospiritual. In the second, by means of a series of clinical vignettes, he provides the groupworker with practical and helpful techniques for facilitating each of these contexts and perspectives.

Working More Creatively with Groups is well known to countless social workers, psychologists and community workers. This new edition not only provides a basic guide to groupwork but also shows how to move on to more in-depth and intensive work.

Jarlath F. Benson is a psychotherapist working in private practice in Belfast and London.

Working More Creatively with Groups

Second edition

Jarlath F. Benson

Routledge
Taylor & Francis Group

LONDON AND NEW YORK

First published 1987
by Tavistock Publications Ltd

Reprinted 1991, 1993, 1995, 1996 and 1997
by Routledge

Second edition published 2001
by Routledge
2 Park Square, Milton Park, Abingdon, Oxon, OX14 4RN

Simultaneously published in the USA and Canada
by Routledge
270 Madison Avenue, New York, NY0016

Reprinted 2004, 2005 (twice), 2006

Routledge is an imprint of the Taylor & Francis Group, an informa business

© 1987, 2001 Jarlath F. Benson

Typeset in Sabon and Gill Sans by RefineCatch Limited,
Bungay, Suffolk
Printed and bound in Great Britain by MPG Books Ltd,
Bodmin, Cornwall

British Library Cataloguing in Publication Data
A catalogue record for this book is available from the British Library

Library of Congress Cataloging in Publication Data
Benson, Jarlath F.
  Working more creatively with groups/Jarlath F. Benson – 2nd ed.
    p. cm.
  Includes bibliographical references and index.
1. Group Counseling. I. Title.
  BF637.C6B37   2000
  158'.35 – dc21   00–32300

ISBN 10: 0–415–23037–3 (hbk)
ISBN 10: 0–415–23038–1 (pbk)
ISBN 13: 978–0–415–23037–7 (hbk)
ISBN 13: 978–0–415–23038–4 (pbk)

For Judy who really does make it all worthwhile

Contents

Acknowledgements

Many people have contributed to the making of this book and I have acknowledged them in the first edition. Of those important people Bill Schwarz and Fr. Miceal O'Regan O.P. have sadly passed away and I miss them very much. Since I wrote the first edition I trained as a group analyst with the Institute of Group Analysis who set up a training course in Dublin. This was an invaluable albeit painful experience and I wish to thank the training team particularly my group analyst Tom Hamrogue for their insight and encouragement.

My wife Judy Kennedy continues to be an enduring source of inspiration as do my daughters Emer, Orla and Lia. They constitute my primary group and have provided profound love, insight, practice and learning over the years.

The Institute of Psychosynthesis in London where I have taught since 1990 has provided me with many fine colleagues who have helped me distill my ideas and develop my practice. To them I offer thanks and deep respect. Sincere thanks and gratitude again go to Joan and Roger Evans and in particular to my dear friend Danielle Roex who is probably one of the finest and most sensitive group-workers around.

Finally I wish to thank all my readers who have let me know in so many ways over the years how helpful and encouraging they have found this book. It has been immensely gratifying to hear how people have valued the first edition and how it has accompanied them on their first tentative steps into groupwork.

Jarlath F. Benson
June 2000

Introduction

Many of the problems and questions of group life can be dealt with in one of two ways – either by giving prescription and information or by creating opportunities in which personal and direct experience itself reveals meaning and suggests resolution. For example, a leader can respond to a new and anxious group where members are asking endless questions:

- Let's not ask any more questions for now and find something to do together.
  or
- I think the answer to your question is this. . . .

Here is another way:

- I notice that many of you are asking a lot of questions today. What is it like for you that you don't know all the answers about this group?

The first answers can deal with the situation but may miss or avoid what is really happening. By contrast the third answer endeavours to lead the enquirer into his own experience, open up, and involve him in the real nature of his need to know. From such experience and awareness of events may emerge meaning and more suitable ways of handling situations in groups.

In essence this is the central thesis and belief advanced in this book: that it is desirable, more respectful, and more creative to involve the whole person in interaction and enquiry and makes most sense to involve the group in its own development, learning, and resolution.

The need for context

The first thing that one needs is a context, a frame of reference which informs and disciplines, and so I want to put forward some of the principles which underpin and guide my own approach to working with groups.

Such a context was not immediately evident when I first started working with groups. As a newcomer to the groupwork scene I might have been excused for feeling that I would be more at home in a martian supermarket. Knowing what type of groups there were, which theory to choose, how to discriminate between technologies, selecting appropriate methods for use in a particular situation appeared to me to require the wisdom of Solomon. I felt very confused and uncertain as to what approach or line was best to take, so what I did was to try a little bit of everything. I operated on the principle – if it works use it, if it doesn't, junk it!

As it turned out, this proved not to be such a bad idea as it might first appear. I experimented, both as member and practitioner with various brands and schools of groupwork and adapted their insights and techniques to fit my particular circumstances. I read widely and was not afraid to raid other fields and disciplines for ideas or tools which I could use. I plagiarized, improvised, and synthesized and always allowed practice to determine what was true. Gradually out of this intensely pragmatic approach there began to emerge a rationale and recurrent working principles which I found could 'travel' and could provide me with a framework for intervening in a wide variety of group environments. Here are some of the more important of these principles:

- Group experience is fundamental
- The group provides consistency and predictability
- The group is organic and natural
- The group is an energetic experience
- The 'here and now' is important
- The 'hidden' must be made visible
- Experience in the group is multi-dimensional
- There is an organizing principle in the group

I want to make some brief statements about these principles in turn.

Group experience is fundamental

At birth we are introduced into our first, small, and intensely personal group, called the family. This group offers the new human being protection and identity. It also offers an opportunity to develop and individuate from the mass experience of humanity as well as providing a qualitative aspect to life.

In its turn the family is dependent for its survival, identity, beliefs, and behaviour on membership of a wide range of formal and informal groups in the larger society – school, church, political, friendship, interest, leisure, and work groups. So from birth we are enlisted in, and gradually committed to, group living in a variety of forms.

Some areas of group influence

• Learning	• Habits
• Attitudes	• Achievement and Performance
• Values	• Mental and emotional well-being

Here are some of the practice applications of this first principle that we will look at in later chapters.

- Developing a sense of identity, support, belonging
- Negotiating the beginning stage of work
- Establishing cohesion, trust, interdependence
- Developing norms, values, rules
- Identifying and meeting individual and group needs

The group provides consistency and predictability

Because of the sheer scope and mass of human experience, group relationships are vital in the birth, nurturing, and maturing of the individual's sense of self. Modern writers in the field believe, like Hargreaves,[1] that the 'self arises from the social experience of interacting with others'. Bernard Davies[2] is even more explicit.

Interaction with other selves is not merely a process which releases the 'core' features and attributes of a person. The individual 'is actually *constructed* in relations with others'. Interaction among humans is what 'defines' and 'creates' a person's experience of self.

But interaction does not occur in a vacuum. Individuals need to engage in interaction frequently, and over a period of time if these social interactions are to become patterned and if expectations concerning each other's behaviour are to develop. Without the *consistency* and *predictability* which comes with patterned and regular interaction, the self which emerges from such transactions is weak, diffuse, and prone to chaos, as anyone who has worked with highly disturbed children, or psychiatric patients, can attest.

The function of the group

And this is where the experience of group is so important. The group is a unique way of transforming or stepping down the mass potential and chaos of undifferentiated human contact into manageable units of predictable and consistent interaction, shared experience, and normative behaviour within which the self can arise. The group provides the context within which socialization and the formation and development of self occurs. Without the group the individual cannot emerge from mass humanity and without the individual the group is just another amorphous mass of living matter.

Practice applications

- Developing a sense of identity and belonging (page 88)
- Establishing cohesion and trust (page 101)
- Making contracts, using power and authority (page 106)
- Creating context, boundary, structure (page 96)
- Identifying and working with roles (page 192)
- Developing norms and values (page 95)

The group is organic and natural

There are a bewildering number of definitions of what a group is, and as a result, there seem to be many apparently conflicting definitions. The reason for this is that an author often selects the relations or properties that are of special importance in his work and then posits these as the criteria for group existence. We can, however, identify a list of attributes that various theorists agree are especially important features of groups.[3]

Key concepts

- A set of people engage in frequent interaction
- They identify with one another
- They are defined by others as a group
- They share beliefs, values, and norms about areas of common interest
- They define themselves as a group
- They come together to work on common tasks and for agreed purposes

What emerges from this list are three very important characteristics of a group:

- There are parts
- There is relationship between the parts
- There is an organizing principle

In other words a group is organic and intentional and not just some random experience.

People come together in a group to satisfy some common need or interest that can be expressed as the group purpose. A network of social relationships is generated within which members accept or reject each other and engage in selected activities. As they do so, *roles* become established and *values* and norms of behaviour emerge, through which individuals can modify and influence each other over time.

This is the understanding I have in mind whenever future reference is made in this book to a group. I am talking about a group as a natural and purposeful experience, involving people in mutual interaction and acceptance, over a period of time, and not just any arbitrary massing of people, a bus queue or shoppers in a supermarket.

Practice applicatons

- Negotiating beginnings, middles, and ends (page 184)
- Learning how to pace, maintain individual and collective action (page 160)
- Clarifying purpose and goals (page 99)
- Developing interaction and 'right relationship' (page 168)
- Understanding individual and collective behaviour (page 65)

The group is an energetic experience

Individual and group experience and interaction change in condition and quality over time. Because the group is organic and natural there is an ebb and flow that we can call process. This group process can be emotionally and physically felt and the worker should aim to develop skills of working with process in order to facilitate group interaction and goal achievement. In particular you will need to learn to work with the two core experiences of group life – the urge to be separate and the need to belong. Let me explain.

The momentum to differentiate from mass consciousness is experienced by the individual as a need to detach and separate (initially from 'mother'). This drive towards independence is clearly beneficial as it widens horizons, provides new learning situations, and opens up contact with an ever-decreasing range of novel objects and situations.

The urge to detach gives rise to one dimension of the experience of self which is a uniquely personal one of distinction, aloneness, and separation. And yet, at the very least human beings are dependent on each other for survival and identity. So there is a contrary pull back towards mass, attachment, dependence, and being a part of something bigger than self. This attachment process refers to one of the simplest and yet most fundamental elements in social behaviour – the tendency to seek the proximity of other members of the species. Again this is a relatively clear-cut principle, occurring almost universally in animals as well as in man. It gives rise to the other dimension of the self – the need to be dependent and in relationship with others. As we will see in Chapter 3, it is the tension generated between these two poles of human experience – the urge to be separate and the need to be attached – which is the drive mechanism for movement and growth in groups.

Each participant in a group experience, and every group if it is to survive and evolve, has to reconcile the urge to separate with the need to be attached. Failure to resolve or even recognize these fundamental human drives results in warped and anti-human experience in groups and gives rise to the fears and anxieties many people express about involvement in collective situations. Chapters 4 to 8 provide ideas and suggestions to help you work with these ideas in practice.

Practice applications

- Understanding and managing behaviour at beginning, middle, and end of group (page 79)
- Working with conflict, tiredness, boredom, being stuck (page 192)
- Teaching process analysis (page 189)
- Teaching group maintenance skills (page 183)
- Balancing individual and group needs (page 71)
- Co-operating with and facilitating love and will energies (page 76)

The importance of the 'here and now'

Individual and group experience and interaction is continuously unfolding in the present tense of group life. Because of the 'nowness' of process, every experience is open to change and development. While this means that I tend to focus primarily on what is happening 'here and now' in the group for each member, it does not mean that I exclude reflexive or historical perspectives. There are many times and situations where exploration of past experience or 'out-of-group' experience is necessary as a way of helping members understand and deal with present time concerns in the group.

But there are other times when it is necessary to attend to the quality of group experience, the levels of trust, hostility, silence, superficiality, and so on if the group is to progress towards its goals. By looking at what is happening in the 'here and now' situation you can help group members become aware of their responsibility for their own behaviours and experiences and determine more appropriate options and strategies. Asking questions like:

- How are you feeling now?
- What is happening in the group now?
- What do you want now?
- What does this behaviour experience mean for us/you?

has the powerful effect of focusing members' attention in the session. In this way it is possible to utilize and build on the present behaviours and experience of members in the group.

Practice applications

- Problem solving and decision making (page 115)
- Helping members make choices (page 142)
- Improving communication and interaction (page 131)
- Helping members be more authentic (page 173)
- Developing a sense of personal power and self-responsibility in members (page 183)
- Emphasizing the importance of themes and patterns in collective behaviour (page 79)

Making the 'hidden' visible

In groups people play 'games' with each other in order to produce certain responses which will reinforce and confirm their beliefs about themselves. These 'games' are also a way of dealing with situations and interactions which might prove fearful, anxious, or involve anger, dependency, helplessness, and aloneness. The result is to distort reality and perception and inhibit creativity and authenticity.

Part of your job as leader is to engage people in the business of making explicit the hidden messages in communications within the group so as to reveal and open up for resolution the problems and difficulties faced by members. Sometimes these messages and feelings are unconscious – members are unaware of what they are feeling or doing in certain situations and at these times a lot of work has to go into uncovering individual and group dynamics in order to create insight and understanding and work more effectively.

Making hidden thoughts, feelings, and desires visible so as to facilitate interaction and activity is one of the most important and frequent tasks you will be called on to perform in the group and Chapters 4 to 8 contain much that will help you with this task.

Experience in the group is multi-dimensional

To be more accurate I should say that each group member operates or experiences the world on a number of different levels and the coming together of people can give an aggregate level or dimension of experience in a group. It is possible to talk about these levels as if they were separate, since each has different functions and requirements. They each need to be addressed if the individual and group experience is to be complete and meaningful. At the physical level members are sensitive to light, heat, cold, noise, hunger, the type of seating, the need for movement, activity, and the like. All these factors have a major influence on the ability of members to participate and on the quality of interaction. It is important that you recognize people's needs at the physical level and respond accordingly.

At the emotional level members find that they have various feelings about the work, the leader, and each other which can enhance, but more often interrupt proceedings. Again, it is essential that you are able to recognize this, and provide ways and means of channelling and transforming emotional energy if your group is not to get stuck or torn apart by violent and conflictual feelings.

There is an intellectual level of experience at which members need to know the objectives and purpose of the group, understand, and comprehend different aspects of the work and generally hold opinions, beliefs, and attitudes. Much of your work in the group at this level will be geared to helping members generate ideas, formulate plans, anticipate consequences, and understand the meaning of their actions.

It is important to be able to work at these different levels and Chapters 4 to 8 give clear suggestions and hints for practice at various stages of the group's development. In Chapters 9 and 10 I offer ideas and guidelines which will help you move from one mode of experience to another. This is particularly useful when working with people who are not very verbally proficient or who find it hard to conceptualize. I have talked a little about Maslow's ideas regarding human needs in Chapter 3 and this will give you a context within which you can understand the importance of the physical, emotional, and intellectual levels of individual and group experience. If you want to read more about the influence of these three aspects at the level of individual personality some of the psychosynthesis books are very interesting and have ideas that transfer naturally to group settings.[4]

There is an organizing principle in the group

What brings a number of individuals together to form a group is their belief and hope that the group can offer means of satisfying their particular needs. This belief and hope is institutionalized in the 'group purpose' and it is this purpose which I see as the principle of organization in any group. Without a purpose the group has no meaning or relevance and is a sterile, usually chaotic experience. Purpose engages members at the level of will to plan objectives and strategies, to organize, make choices, and execute in action. Purpose creates boundary, structure, parameter and really provides the conditions and circumstances within which the other principles referred to, can operate.

A slightly different perspective on purpose is yielded by my use of the word 'vision'. The concept of vision recurs continually throughout this work and refers to the range of possibilities that a group can open up for its members. I use the notion of vision to convey a deeper sense of the group purpose. Vision points to the potential inherent in collective action and indicates what we may be if we choose accordingly. Vision sustains the group through the dark and stormy periods of its life when it is all too easy for members to slip into despair and hopelessness. Vision provides the values and beliefs by which group members decide to live and work together. Of course the vision of possibility indicated in a particular group must be incarnated in everyday group experience if it is not to remain at an abstract and intangible level.

Together vision and its more solid manifestation, purpose, provide a 'centre' or organizing principle in the group which becomes more real and strong as it is used. Initially this vision or purpose is carried by the worker for members only until such time as they can begin to develop and formulate their own personal vision of what the group means. This theme is more fully developed in Chapter 8 so that it is only relevant here to emphasize the importance of ensuring that you can clearly articulate why it is that you believe a group can help these particular people at this time.

A definition

Putting all these principles together, it is possible to see now what the context for practice is and even make a clear statement about what is meant by groupwork practice:

> Groupwork practice refers to the conscious, disciplined, and systematic use of knowledge about the processes of collective human interaction, in order to intervene in an informed way, or promote some desired objective in a group setting. In the sense that it is used in this book, groupwork practice is a *helping process designed to correspond to specific instances of individual and group need, based on a view of man as in constant interaction and relationship with others.* Groupwork is a productive, healthy, and creative experience, carried out on the basis of *explicit agreements,* openly pursued and clearly arrived at, about the purpose and task of the group, rights, and responsibilities of members.

Chapter 1

How to plan the group

The importance of planning cannot be emphasized enough – as our traditional folk wisdom shows. Foresight and organization are the basis of many of our favourite proverbs: 'Look before you leap', 'A stitch in time saves nine', 'Prevention is better than cure', and so on.

Yet despite the abundance and richness of these traditional insights many groups still fail to get off the ground or splutter into anonymity after a few sessions, due simply to the fact that not enough attention was given, before the group even started, to its planning and organization. There are many reasons for this. From time to time, I still come across the 'it'll be all right on the day' types or the leaders who believe that planning the group is manipulative or will detract from the involvement of members. Even some who do conscientiously try to organize their thinking about their reasons and purposes for using groupwork, often generate goals and objectives for a group that are unrealistic or grandiose. Much of the conflict and hostility which can then ensue in those groups is simply a product of the leaders' resentment and frustration with members who won't seem to 'work', and members' anger and confusion about the discrepancy between what they are capable of, or willing to do, and what is expected of them.

Before we go on to look at some procedures for planning the group let me say a bit more about why it is important to plan.

Why plan a group?

Whatever their ages, interests, or concerns, individual members come to the group with their own perception of what they want, or do not want from the experience. As the group develops, a common perception of need or interest emerges, which may or may not be compatible with the wants and desires of members (see page 65). At some point both individual and group perceptions of needs and goals will be tested against the worker's perception of the group purpose.

As Whitaker says, if a worker is not clear in his mind about the sort of group he wishes to conduct, 'he will almost inevitably present mixed cues and signals to the group'.[1] Douglas goes even further. A group leader has got to have a 'reasonable certainty about what he intends to do'.[2] Particularly where a group leader is working with suspicious, disbelieving, or hostile clients, 'if his own ideas and values are hazy then he will not be convincing'.[3]

But there are other reasons for planning a group:

- To assess the degree of need and plan a response
- To determine if groupwork is appropriate in the circumstances
- To clarify the purpose of the group
- To focus on members' needs
- To identify specific outcomes
- To determine how these will be achieved. (A plan is the means employed to achieve particular ends or outcomes.)
- To help potential members see the group as a means of meeting their needs
- To pinpoint difficulties or obstacles and develop coping strategies
- To identify resources
- To clarify roles, expectations, tasks of workers and members

---

Clearly we could extend this list. The point is that leaders who start groups without being clear about their reasons for using groupwork, without adequate planning, or whose desired outcomes are vague are bound for trouble. In my introduction I said that my own style of groupwork was concerned with the 'here and now' of individual and group experience. This does not mean that I walk into a group without having considered why I am there, what I can or cannot offer, or without having done some preparation to help group members use a particular experience or activity to achieve an agreed objective.

My own experience is that the ability to work creatively and spontaneously in a group and use the unexpected incidents that frequently occur, is based on a solid foundation of advance planning and consideration. In architecture there is a dictum, 'Form follows function', and this is good advice for group workers. We need to spend time identifying the function of the group in order to arrive at the most appropriate form for realizing our purposes.

A guide to planning

If Douglas is right that a group leader ought to have a 'reasonable certainty about what he intends to do' then we need to look at what activities the leader engages in to acquire this conviction. In the following sections I want to explore in some detail what I consider are the major planning activities of the group leader. My intention is not to suggest that planning a group is an operation which is absolutely and definitive or precludes negotiation and agreement with members. The focus throughout is on the worker and what he can do before the first session to help the group become more effective. But first let us ask a question:

> Is planning for an existent group different from planning for a group convened by the leader?

There are two ways in which a worker can engage with a group. Either he can convene the group himself or he can be invited or required to work with an already existing group.

If a leader works with an existent group he has not convened, the only difference this makes to the planning process is that:

- The group leader does not select group members. They are already selected
- He does not determine the goals or purposes of the group though he may help to clarify them
- He may have his role prescribed though he may be free within limits to perform it as he sees fit
- The programme may be prescribed although the group leader may have some control over content

---

With these constraints in mind I want to suggest a method which can apply to the planning of any group whether it already exists or has yet to be formed. There are six stages in this formulation:

- Researching and justifying the need for groupwork
- Attending to membership
- Programming the group
- Leading the group
- Presenting the group
- Planning the first session

The first three stages will be discussed now and the final three explored in the next chapter.

Researching and justifying the need for groupwork

There are a number of steps in this phase of planning.

Becoming aware of the problem

The first point to consider is *how the demand* for group service or membership *comes to your attention*. Is it a *request* from an already existing group for help with, let's say, programme design; from a colleague who wants you to work with some of the children on his caseload because 'you are good with kids', or from a woman you know who is socially isolated and wants to join a group to make friends? Perhaps the provision of a group service is a *requirement* of your job. You may be expected to reach out to young people through groupwork or required to encourage and facilitate the work of community action groups. Is the idea of groupwork a *response* on your part to emerging client needs or recognized themes in team, office, agency workload? Considering how the demand for groupwork comes to your attention is important because it raises some important points:

- Who makes the application?
- For whom?
- Why?
- What do they want?
- What do the beneficiaries of the group service actually need?

If you think for a moment you will realize that there are many people who did not originally request help but who are now receiving it. A topical example of this is the current debate in IT (Intermediate Treatment) circles about the 'net-widening' effect of inclusion in IT groups – on children and adolescents who have not appeared before a court. These youngsters are encouraged to join groups because they are considered to be at risk or in need of supervision and support. Much money, resource, and time may be invested in these groups and it is arguable whether the outlay is justifiable in terms of what these young people really require, and the potential for initiating them into a deviant career.

Often such groups are run by people whose full-time occupation is to work with young people and occasionally it can happen that the demand for a group service represents more the needs of workers or an organization to maintain its grant-aid from the local authority, than it does the real needs of potential group members.

In other circumstances people can ask for help with no real understanding of an agency's services or obligations and then find themselves caught up in a programme they are unwilling to be involved in. The point is this, by carefully and thoughtfully assessing how and why you became aware of a particular demand for a group service you can:

- Begin to establish the motivations of yourself and colleagues to offer a service
- Decide that there really is a need that can be met by group-work and which justifies time, resource, and expenditure
- Gather preliminary information about possible goals for a group
- Make it easier for people to participate in relevant pro-grammes
- Highlight the range and functions of agency provisions and the consequences of involvement

Considering the proposal and testing alternatives

Having established that a social situation exists which might prove amenable to groupwork intervention, the next step is to consider if groupwork is in fact the desired or most appropriate response. Ask questions like:

- Is there a clearly demonstrable group need or problem?
- Does a shared need or problem exist among enough people to warrant groupwork?
- Can I identify a common aim which is likely to get agreement?
- Can groupwork really achieve gains for these potential members?
- What sort of gains?
- What special properties of the group do I wish to make use of?
- Are potential members likely to see the group as relevant and helpful?
- Will the group damage or label or stigmatize any member?
- Is there another medium or form of intervention that can achieve the desired outcome as well as the group?
- Why is the group setting more effective than the one-to-one setting?
- Can I make reasonable estimates of time involved, programme, cost?
- Can I get agency approval for the group in terms of use of time, finance, resource?

From the answers to these questions I try to establish that there is a need which is shared by people, is best met by working in a group, and that I can contribute in some way to this need. I find it useful to identify a general aim for the group such as:

- Providing social activity for isolated people.
- Helping a community group clarify its goals.
- Providing emotional support for depressed men and women.

Having a general aim for the group focuses thinking and makes it easier to locate relevant literature or talk to other group leaders who have worked in this area, in order to obtain a better understanding of the needs of the group and learn about more effective and appropriate ways of working. However, aims are often stated in such general terms that it is not possible to evaluate whether they have been achieved or not. Subsequently I try to break aims down into narrower, more specific goals or objectives. This goal setting is important because:

- Goals motivate behaviour. An *individual goal* is the reason why a member joins a group. A *group goal* is a future state of affairs desired by enough members of the group to motivate them working towards its achievement
- Goals are guides for action. Goals indicate to worker and members, the tasks that must be performed, the behaviours and processes of interaction that must be engaged in if the goal is to be achieved.
- Goals are a way of attaining agreement and resolving conflict.
- Goals are a way of evaluating the effectiveness of group procedures. Without goals there is nothing to evaluate (see page 294).

Examples of goals in a group might be:

- To help John improve his conversational skills.
- To prevent children going into care.
- To clarify role requirements in the team.

Some goals, which might refer to the worker's desired outcomes can be specified at this stage; other goals require the approval and adoption by members and must be negotiated in the group itself. Louis Lowy suggests a number of principles that should be adhered to by the group leader when identifying goals for the group.[4]

- Worker goals should be based on assessment of group members and stage of group development.
- Goals should be stated in behavioural terms.
- Goals should refer to state of improved functioning of members and group.
- Goals should be realistic and achievable.
- Goals should be prioritized.
- Goal formation should be a shared process involving members and worker.

By pinpointing some goals at this stage you can begin to see if, how, and why groupwork is an appropriate method to use in a particular setting.

Justifying the group

The final area of importance in this research phase of group planning concerns the relationship of the group to the agency, institution, or community of which it is a part. Whitaker suggests that, 'there are many settings in which it is not prudent to undertake groupwork until after one has thoroughly explored one's plans with one's colleagues'.[5] There are good reasons for this.

Professionals are often deeply suspicious of groups, sometimes even hostile. I have worked with many who have been exposed to groupwork 'teaching' on their training courses, which has left them embittered and cynical because of what they regard as the manipulativeness of group workers, the potential for damaging group experience, or the impenetrable mystique which surrounds groupwork. Parsloe talks about the 'shared fantasy amongst social workers about what goes on in groups', and suggests that some elements of this fantasy are believed to be that the group leader never breaks a silence, seldom speaks, is apparently always free from anxiety, and able to expose the raw feelings of an individual or the group, at a stroke.[6]

No doubt some professionals have experienced this sort of groupwork and it creates in them a wish to protect their clients from similar experiences. It is important to reassure these workers, if you can; and discuss with them how you see the group and what it can offer members in terms of gains. Unless you deal with colleagues' reservations or mixed feeling about groups you can find that they pass their fears onto clients; they are dilatory in making referrals to you or they just simply refuse to co-operate.

One way of securing the support of colleagues is to demonstrate to them that the involvement of clients in a group can actually contribute to and enhance their work. To do this you should determine what the objectives of the agency or institution are in respect of the potential group members. Ensure that the general aim and the goals for your group are compatible with agency objectives and you are not proposing to work in an area that is the concern of another organization (social worker intending to teach children literacy and numeracy skills, youth worker offering a therapy group for depressed youngsters). This is important because crossing professional boundaries or working in grey areas can undermine your credibility and expose you to charges that the proposal is irrelevant to the remit of the agency and cannot justify resource and expenditure.

You should identify the agency's actual operational concerns in relation to potential group members and establish what the priorities are. Try to work out the contribution your group can make to the service being offered by the agency and pinpoint where the group will enhance, back-up, or confirm the work of colleagues.

It is worth putting this information on paper even though at this stage it may represent only brief outline thinking about the proposed group, its aims, and contribution to agency delivery of service. Here is part of an actual outline proposal from my own work which illustrates thinking at this stage.

EXAMPLE

Outline plan for working with depressed women on a group therapy basis. A definition of problem and focus of work: A number of women have been identified on existing casework loads by individual caseworkers as in need of involvement in a therapeutic peer group, which would help them deal with their depressive feelings.

The background of these women could be summarized as follows:

- Single parent and usually with child management difficulties.
- A number of women have children on the NAI register (non-accidental injury register: a list of children abused by parents and held by the social services).
- Marked degree of social isolation due to poor family relationships, lack of social support, etc.
- Poor housing conditions, low income.

Against this background the following responses have been observed in the women:

- A perception of self as of low value and worth.
- An ineffective or inadequate presentation and use of self.
- An inability or reluctance to assume an appropriate degree of responsibility for their selves and their behaviour.

These three responses would appear to produce problematic behaviour such as depression, communication and relationship problems, poor motivation, poor child management.

Possible goals for group

- To begin to relieve the distress that these women are obviously experiencing by offering a group support.
- To bring together women who live in the same neighbourhood in order to jointly tackle problems encountered in their mutual experience.
- To help the women work on what they identify as the painful and distressing areas of their life.
- To help the women develop strategies for dealing more effectively with distress and depression.

Why a group?

- The women all come from the same neighbourhood although only one or two know each other.
- They have similar problems: single parents, child management difficulties, depression, social isolation.
- The group can offer companionship, support, encouragement to work on depression, feedback, opportunities to make relationships.
- The women would be willing to attend the group.
- The group offers the caseworker another therapeutic option, assessment facilities, as well as providing additional monitoring of high-risk cases.

An outline like this is not a final plan with estimates of cost, resource, programme details, methodology, and worker's role, clearly delineated. It is merely a proposal which helps your colleagues and managers understand more about your project, enables them to express their views and feel involved. Whitaker believes that a group is more likely to be successful if colleagues 'accept and support its aims and general procedures and value its potential contribution to the shared goals of the organization or institution'.[7] With an outline like this you can ask for permission to gather referrals, secure a promise of resources and funding, and move to the next phase of planning. Even in situations where you do not have to persuade colleagues or superiors of the need for groupwork you should still commit early thoughts to paper.

Attending to membership

The constituency of group membership can exercise a powerful effect on the interaction that ensues and can facilitate or inhibit the progress of the group towards the goals for which it was formed. Whether you form a group for the first time or are working with an existent group it is important to pay attention to the implications of membership for group effectiveness (see page 26).

Knowing something about who is in the group and why, can help you:

- Identify individual motivations and needs
- Plan individual goals, where appropriate
- Formulate group goals
- Select members, where appropriate
- Assess the likely effect of members on each other
- Anticipate unhelpful behaviour and interaction
- Encourage facilitative behaviour and interaction
- Plan a relevant programme
- Pitch the programme at a suitable level
- Suggest a particular leadership style

Recruitment

Some workers take an active part in recruiting and selecting members for the group. There is general agreement that decisions about size and potential membership in such groups are based on:

- The agency's goals and expectations of the group.
- The worker's goals for the group.
- The needs and goals of potential members.
- Group goals that are likely to emerge over time.

Another widely accepted principle is that groups should be *similar* enough to ensure commonality of need and compatibility but *disparate* enough to ensure that members will be stimulating and useful to each other. Some leaders will select particular individuals for a group because of their similarity or disparity on certain *descriptive* and *behavioural* attributes. Descriptive attributes, 'classify an individual as to age, sex, marital status, occupation, or other "positions" he may be said to occupy', while behavioural attributes, 'describe the way an individual acts or can be expected to act based on his past performance'.

Paradise and Daniels list eighteen descriptive and behavioural attributes they take into consideration when selecting children for group membership.[8] These attributes include: need to belong to the group, ability to communicate, ability to tolerate behavioural differences, level of dependency, level of aggression, ability to delay gratification, age, sex, and socio-economic status.

Bertcher and Maple suggest that a group is more effective if members have *similar descriptive attitudes* as this encourages cohesion, interactiveness, and compatibility, and *disparate behavioural attributes* because this increases 'the behavioural repertoire that will be useful to the group' and fosters interest and responsiveness.[9]

Groups will not be effective if there is:

- Too much compatibility – can become 'samey' and stagnant
- Too much or too little stress
- Not enough creativity or novelty
- Negative or dissenting sub-groups

Important descriptive attributes group leaders often consider are:

- *Age and developmental level:* When working with children and young people I tend to keep to a narrow age band – usually two years between oldest and youngest – in order to capitalize on similar interests and abilities when programming and making decisions. Often an older but emotionally less developed child can be placed in a younger age group where he can feel more comfortable. In adult groups a wider age-spread is more usual and can be valuable to teach younger adults from the experience of older adults. These older members can also learn from younger members how to resolve problems or difficulties left over from an earlier stage.

- *Sex*: While my own preference is to work with mixed sex groups where possible, as being more normal in relation to social life, there are situations where it can be more advantageous to work in single-sex groups. For example my experience with groups of eight- to ten-year-old and eleven- to thirteen-year-old children is that they tend to split into sub-groups along sex lines and it can be very hard to develop cohesion particularly where the purpose of the group is to focus on a task. It is often just better to work in a single-sex group with these age-sets. I find that five- to seven-year-olds and fourteen- to seventeen-year-olds can better manage the inter-sex relationships in a group and this can be used to effect. With some adult groups, women's consciousness raising groups, groups who explore sexual issues, or whose purpose is to express the trauma of rape, incest, or sexual assault, there may be good reasons to work in single-sex setting where the presence of members of the opposite sex would be embarrassing, provocative, or counter-productive.

- *Geographical proximity*: In some circumstances leaders like to work with people from the same neighbourhood as a way of consolidating and transferring the learning that goes on in the group setting to the domestic environment. Many IT workers seek to work with adolescent peer groups as a way of countering deviant norms, believing the groups if modified will be more resistant to the delinquent sub-culture than lone individuals. Where people join groups to deal with the problems created by social isolation it makes sense to work with them if they all live in a neighbourhood where they can continue contact between meetings.

  In other instances geographical proximity can be a disadvantage. When confidentiality is important, as in a therapeutic group, members' relationships, previous knowledge of each other, or even just knowing that another member lives in the same estate can be an impediment to self-expression and the development of trust. My experience is that confidentiality is more likely to break down in groups where members are drawn from the same vicinity, for obvious reasons.

Behavioural attributes that are considered important by many leaders are:

- *Ability to communicate*: If a potential member finds it hard to verbalize his feelings and thoughts it could be damaging to him and inhibitive of the group to place him in a setting where the major activity is intended to be discussion. He may require a group more suited to his ability and level of communication.

- *Degree of disturbance*: This has to be carefully assessed in treatment contexts if individuals are not to be scapegoated or provoked and the group is not to be severely impeded or held up.
- *Motivation to work or join in group activity*: If the group is to be successful it is important to be able to gauge how willing each individual is to be in the group and involve himself in its work. In many groups members attend reluctantly, to appease parents, social workers, probation officers, or authority figures; such groups rarely work.
- *Ability to relate to others*: It is important to know that an individual is able to relate to others even minimally, because of the interpersonal nature of the group. Paradise and Daniels point out four aspects of this variable.[10]

1 How *sensitive* is the individual to the feelings and behaviour of other people?

2 Does the individual have adequate defence mechanisms to fall back on in adversity?

3 How able is the individual to *delay gratification* particularly in a setting where shared experience is emphasized?

4 *How dependent* is an individual in relationships?

There is an alternative view to the active recruitment and selection of members by the group leader. Some other leaders simply form the group by taking whoever is available at the time and responsive to the stated group goal. Tropp states that, 'there is no point in trying to determine what combination of particular individual characteristics would make the most effective group composition.'[10] He believes that it is 'undesirable to collect all this data' because it is not possible to predict future group behaviour of an individual and because, 'it creates a contaminating process whereby the members become aware of the leader's prior knowledge and judgements about them', and tend to behave in ways that fulfil these expectations.[11] All that needs to be known is that there is commonalty of need and that no member 'is going to be clearly harmful to or harmed by the group experience.'[12]

This is a viewpoint on recruitment that I have a lot of sympathy with. When I first started working with groups I used to ask for referrals that gave me information on such variables as age, sex, intelligence, language ability, degree of disturbance, sociability, and so on. I then rigorously combed these referrals trying to create the optimum combination of members for the group. I have been repeatedly surprised when individuals did not behave as was predicted from the referral. Now I am more cautious about information on a potential group member that may have been gleaned from a formal one-to-one setting. Even when I know information comes from seeing the individual in the collectivity of school, family, or institution I am aware that the spontaneity, informality, and egalitarian nature of the group setting can release different and previously unseen qualities in the person which can make reliance solely on *historical* factors for selection unwise.

Sometimes there are situations in which there is a commonalty of need but there are such marked differences that it is important to think carefully about their possible consequences. These may be differences of race, religion, or political affiliation, known rivalries and tensions which normally would make it very difficult for the group to work. On these occasions I check with the potential members beforehand if they feel that these differences will affect them adversely but usually I find that people's need for the group service is sufficient to overcome these apparent barriers. Infrequently a potential member will refuse to join because of such factors but only rarely in my experience have these differences disrupted a group. As far as possible I now prefer to let group purpose and the setting I am operating in, determine how members are recruited.

To give an example: there are often occasions in which I will make an offer of a groupwork service to people I have no first hand knowledge of, to deal with a certain need or problem in a particular neighbourhood. In response to a community request I will let it be known that I am forming a group to help addicted youngsters stop glue-sniffing, or provide single parents with social support and contact. In these circumstances I would follow Tropp's suggestions and work with whoever responded to the group objective if it was at all clear that they could benefit by, and contribute to the group experience. The only criterion I would apply after this would be numerical. If too many turn up I suggest either a second group to run concurrently or if this isn't possible I ask members present to decide among themselves the urgency of their need to be in the group, and offer a placement to those who can wait until the first group has ended. This is usually a satisfactory arrangement for all concerned.

While I do not ignore completely what descriptive and behavioural attributes are available I am much more concerned with the needs of individuals to be in the group, and their motivation to be there and to use the experience. To this end it is important to have contact where possible with potential members before the group starts in order to clarify expectations, responsibilities, requirements, and objectives (see 'Presenting the group', page 43).

Structural issues

SIZE

The purposes and needs of the group should determine its size. In a therapy group where the emphasis is on self-disclosure, intimacy, and support, membership would be smaller (eight and under) than in an activity group where a larger membership (up to twelve and often more) would ensure more variety, skills, and resources. An educational group can have more members (up to twenty-five) because there may be more passivity and reliance on a leader or teacher than a work group (under seven) where energy and attention tends to be focused on the doing of certain tasks. Here are some variables to think about when considering size.

- Intimacy
- Support   } Decreases as numbers get larger
- Satisfaction

- Opportunity to participate   } Increases as numbers get smaller
- Consensus

- Personal recognition decreases
- Number of personal relationships increase
- Sub-groups emerge
- More reliance on leader   As numbers
- More need for formal procedures and rules   increase
- Ability to tackle more complex problems develops
- Problem solving takes longer
- More creativity

There is general agreement that an optimum size for a group is seven members.'[13] This is large enough to allow recognition, intimacy, and involvement. In the learning group seven to thirteen seems to work out best while five is a good size for a work group although larger numbers do provide more resource and skills.[14]

FREQUENCY AND NUMBER OF MEETINGS

Again this is something which is determined by group purposes and needs. Generally I find that the deeper I need to go in exploring interpersonal or ego issues the more time is required to build up trust, cohesion, and safety. For individuals to take risks with increasingly private material, the group needs the consistency and predictability that comes with regular and patterned interaction (see page 78). In the more overtly therapeutic group setting I go for weekly meetings held over a six-month period (twenty-five sessions) for adults, or nine months (thirty-six sessions) for children.

For more task-oriented groupwork such as team development, social skills training, or educational groups, I again choose a weekly meeting, but over a shorter time span – anything from six to twelve weeks depending on the availability of time, group needs, and purpose. The reason for this is that there is quite a different emphasis on relationships in the work group than in the therapy group.

Sessions in the therapy context last for three hours. This sounds very long but I find that this permits a maximum number of group members to participate. Work groups I usually fix at two-and-a-half hours and very occasionally two hours. I almost never work a shorter session. Many other leaders prefer to have a session lasting between one and two hours because they are afraid that members will get bored or tired with a longer session. In my experience group members do respond to the longer sessions, and boredom or tiredness when they occur, become an opportunity to help the group acquire maintenance skills (see page 183).

Flexibility and creativity in the use of managing time is important in most groupwork settings. Weekly and fortnightly meetings sustain the momentum and build up a sense of belonging and commitment as well as the consistency and predictability which is so important if a group is to be healthy and productive. But there are many situations in which it is difficult or inappropriate to use normal time determinants and you may have to be more inventive. In times of crisis – such as sexual assault, death of a relative, sudden mental stress, or terminal illness – an otherwise emotionally destabilizing or hazardous situation can be facilitated by sensitive and flexible groupwork offered within twenty-four to seventy-two hours of 'the cry for help'.[15] One or a number of group sessions lasting from a few hours to a day, a weekend, or spread over some weeks can be offered to crisis victims and their families depending on their need.

In other settings, such as a hospital where patients attending a specialized support group may live in a wide geographical area, occasional one-day or weekend sessions can top up the monthly or (more often) infrequent meetings. Residential and education settings can also respond to more intensive group meeting. In teaching groupwork skills to social work students I will often use a 'ten-hour session'. With work teams where the emphasis is on developing and strengthening work relationships, I always start with a one- or two-day 'nutcracker' intensive as a way of loosening up rigid procedures and ways of thinking before going into the more usual weekly sessions.

Don't be afraid to experiment with the length of session, number and frequency of meetings to suit your group needs. You will find that most people are fairly adaptable and open to new approaches designed to facilitate them.

CLOSED OR OPEN GROUPS

A closed group is one which starts and finishes with the same people and is run for a fixed number of sessions. In an open group members may come and go at different times for various reasons. The time span for the group may be set beforehand or may be left indeterminate.

Programming the group

Programming is a highly skilled part of working in a group. It demands imagination, flexibility, assessment, selection-design, and interventive skills as well as an ability to coordinate human and material resources in a manner which meets the needs of the individual and the group. According to Vinter, the word programme denotes, 'a class of group activities', which 'follow a pattern, unfolding in a rough chronological sequence and sometimes reaching a definite climax or conclusion'.[16] Examples of programme activities would be a game, role-play exercise, group discussion, or making a meal together.

Advantages

Open group	*Closed group*
• Constant modification of group culture	• Consistent and predictable
• Greater variety of resource and skill	• Can be more cohesive and intimate
• Can be more creative, imaginative	• Easier to balance
• Good for work on initiating and terminating relationships	
• Issues of separation, termination, inclusion	
• Issues around change, adaptability	

Disadvantages

Open group	*Closed group*
• Can be more unstable, less predictable	• Tendency to get into conformity and 'group think'
• Lacks depth, intimacy of closed group	• Lacks the range and variety of the open group
• Sub-grouping, cliques, alliances	• Less able to deal with change and adaptability
• Hard to balance	• Limited opportunity to deal with termination issues

Why use programme?

A programme of activities is not an end in itself. Group leaders use programme consciously and carefully in order to influence groups and individuals and achieve specific outcomes. Perhaps the most important reason for using programme is to provide a point of focus – a context for group members to come together. Context creates boundaries and boundaries create rules and structure, consistency and predictability.

As we saw earlier (page 27) without the consistency and predictability that comes from patterned interaction and context, human interaction tends to be weak, diffuse, and anarchic. Children and adults get a sense of who they are and learn by doing and working with others in settings where there is a degree of structure.

When children and adults suffer from relationship difficulties or have a poor image of themselves as a result of missed or absent life-opportunities they can benefit enormously from a carefully structured group experience which aims at rebuilding self-confidence or improving social skills. In other situations where resolution of a problem or task is the reason for the group's existence thoughtful selection of activity by the leader can provide the necessary structure and procedure for helping the group to achieve its objectives. We can list some of the reasons for using programme in the group:

- To provide a medium or context in which members can engage and interact.
- To provide the group with structured experience.
- To influence directly or indirectly the group or individuals.
- To achieve particular results or desired objectives.
- To modify or control undesirable behaviour.
- To facilitate the growth and development of a group.

The important point to remember is that programme should always be related to individual and group needs and goals. The programme is not an end in itself. As a leader you should always be able to say why you are using a certain activity or engaging the group in a particular project.

Creative programme design

Creative programme design is about responding to people in a way that enables them to meet their needs while at the same time helping you achieve group tasks and purposes. To do this the group worker requires certain skills and knowledge. Ross and Bernstein suggest that there are three basic skills needed to purposefully design and use programme.[17]

- Assessment
- Activity selection
- Intervention

ASSESSMENT

There are three components in assessment:

- An individual assessment of the needs of each group member.
- An assessment of the stage of development of the group.
- Identifying the objectives to be achieved.

Chapter 3 contains a detailed account of how to identify individual needs and the stage of group development. All that requires to be said here is that assessment enables the leader to penetrate the welter of needs and problems thrown up by a group and its members, and pinpoint specific and strategic objectives. The important point to remember is that unless compelled to do so members will only attend a group if their expectations and needs are being met. Programme must arise from the needs of members and must be related to their mental and physical capacities as well as the group goals. Clear and accurate assessment, therefore, is the first key to creative programme design. In the early stage of a group I worked with, I asked adolescent boys and girls to engage in a written exercise to rate and prioritize certain desirable personal attributes. To my surprise and frustration they refused to co-operate with my carefully prepared exercise and would proffer no reason other than it was 'stupid' and 'boring'. They would not discuss the matter and got very disruptive when I pressed them. It was after another three or four sessions when I knew them better that they revealed to me that they had major difficulties with reading and writing and were fearful of exposing their impediments in front of relative strangers.

ACTIVITY SELECTION

Having identified individual and group needs and set targets the worker can begin to select or design programme activities which will achieve these targets. However, problems now arise which are familiar to many group leaders. How do you select activities from the vast array of resources available, which will have maximum impact in the desired direction? How do you identify the particular attributes of an activity, that will be relevant to you? How do you then create consciousness among members as to the purpose of the activity?

Robert Vinter has looked at some of these questions and presents a formulation which I find very valuable in analysing, choosing, and modifying programme activities as diverse as football or group discussion.[18] He states that all activities have three elements:

- A *physical field* which is the territory or space, the people, and equipment associated with the activity, e.g. pitch, players, and ball in football.
- *Performance behaviours* which are basic and essential to the activity, e.g. kicking the ball, no handling, tackling opponents.
- *Respondent behaviours* which are evoked by the activity but not essential to it, e.g. hugging and kissing a goal-scorer, cheering, and arguing.

Vinter believes that performance and respondent behaviours can be achieved or modified by informed selection or modification of particular activities. He suggests six features of all activity that are open to modification.

- The rules or procedures for the activity.
- The sources of agents of activity control such as referees, umpires, team captains.
- The degree of physical movement involved.
- Competence levels required to participate.
- The degree of interaction with other people.
- The types of reward associated with the activity.

By altering or fine-tuning these variables, decreasing the level of competence, increasing the degree of physical movement, streamlining the rules, and so on, a group leader can achieve different effects for different members or for the group at critical stages in its development. (See Chapter 10 for suggestions about activities and their appropriateness in group settings.)

INTERVENTION

Intervention is a constellation of skills which require the leader to make ongoing assessment and decisions about how to act in order to encourage, modify, or control behaviour of the group or individuals. This is a very creative and flexible part of the programming process because the leader may need to fine-tune any or all of the activity variables at any stage in the activity.

An important part of the intervention strategy is working out how to create consciousness for group members about the activity and its relevance to their lives. How I try to do this is by having a review of the activity after it has finished. In the review the group and I evaluate:

- The quality of group and member experience.
- Levels of satisfaction.
- Interactions between members.
- What occurred in activity and why?
- What was the purpose of the activity and whether it was accomplished?
- Relevance and significance of activity for individuals and the group.
- What could be improved, modified?
- Where do we go from here?

A review like this need not take very long and can usually be talked through although there are times when it is good to do a written evaluation.

EXAMPLE OF PROGRAMME DESIGN USING THESE VARIABLES

Assessment   I had been working with a group of eight eleven- to thirteen-year-old boys and girls. We were about two months through a nine-month therapy group. Members tended to be quite defensive and solitary. They did not mix well, trust each other, or share much about themselves. I decided to focus on two objectives.

- To encourage and develop trust.
- To encourage the children to co-operate and share.

Programme selection and design I chose guided imaging, drawing, and drama as the components of my programme.

Guided imaging. Conducting the children on a fantasy journey meant I could start with an activity which required no equipment, no performance behaviour, no interaction or movement. I controlled the pace and flow of the activity, there were minimal rules (eyes closed, no noise), and the children did not have to be competent at anything other than making pictures in their imagination in response to prompts from me. The exercise was one which was done alone which meant I started 'where the children were at'.

I chose *drawing* to follow up the fantasy work. Drawing the journey meant that the children would make visible as much as they wished to reveal of their inner activity. The crayons were restricted in number and colour to ensure that the children would have to borrow and share with each other, thereby encouraging interaction.

Depending on the interest generated by the first two stages of the programme I would suggest that we *acted out* one of the children's journeys. This would continue to stimulate the imagination and involve the children in communicating, building action sequences, casting characters, and acting out the final work – all co-operative and shared experience.

Intervention I settled and relaxed the children and then asked them to mentally choose three members of their group to accompany them on a perilous journey to rescue a fairy princess held in a castle owned by a fierce giant.

Choosing three members of their group, ostensibly to guide and advise on dealing with dragons, magic forests, and various hazards:

- Created a (mental) basis for interaction.
- Stressed a positive and helping interaction.
- Created a basis for interaction in actual group reality.
- Provided an experience that the children could share.

After we had completed the fantasy journey I suggested to the children that we should draw details of the experience. I decided to let the children do this individually rather than do a group drawing – the jump from individual imaging to group drawing would have been too big a transition. As the children were drawing I went around looking at the different drawings. I made public comments on the various group members who appeared in the drawings as a way of attracting their attention and generally applauded their exploits, bravery, and wisdom, generating much excitement and interest. The restriction in number and colour of crayons had the desired effect of ensuring that the children talked to each other, negotiated, borrowed, and shared.

It was an easy matter to introduce the idea of acting out a journey and involving group members as themselves, the dragon, the forest, the princess, the hero, and the giant. The drama involved the children in literal performance behaviours but also evoked respondent behaviours in applause, cheering, jeers, and so on. The children were all included in the one activity either as audience or actors. In the short review session afterwards the whole programme was seen as very attractive and popular and, it was felt, had drawn the group closer together. I subsequently repeated the session, building up a more solid foundation upon which the children could communicate and interact more naturally and informally. The whole sequence took two hours.

It is important in the early stages of a group that the leader knows what he is doing and has a programme that can convey this. The scheme we have looked at offers the leader a framework for designing a relevant programme of activities to manage and guide individual and group behaviour irrespective of whether the group is composed of stroke patients, elderly ladies, children, or adults.

Common mistakes in programming

1 Failure to base programme on identified individual or group need.
2 Failure to link programme and group objectives.
3 Programme content or objectives unrealistic (see 1, 2).
4 Programme is too rigid due to over-planning and failure to allow for spontaneous and unexpected incidents and events.
5 Inability to use the unexpected incident to develop programme objectives or take an entirely new course (see 2, 12, 15).
6 Not enough balance between the needs of the person and the requirements of the task (see page 71).
   Programme too little/too much task centred;
                 too little/too much person centred.
7 Programme above or below the mental and physical capacities of members. May show them in a weak or unfavourable light (see 6).

8 Skill and competence levels may be too high or too low, creating frustration, boredom, competition.

9 Programme separates people because of a division of labour, skill, aptitude, interest.

10 Programme may be unimaginative, repetitious, unstimulating (see Chapter 6).

11 Poor or inappropriate selection of activity.

12 Activity becomes an end rather than a means of heightening awareness or experience (see 4, 5, 15).

13 Failure to create consciousness for members around the programme (see 2, 5, 12, 14, 15).

14 Failure to review, evaluate as a way of fine-tuning or redesigning the programme (see 2, 4, 13, 15).

15 Programme can become a way of avoiding work with the group while giving the appearance of industry and business.

Chapter 2

Leading and setting up the group

There is no single, universally applicable style or method of working in a group. Different groups demand different leadership styles and each group will require a variety of behaviours and responses from the leader as it moves through its phases of development towards greater capability and maturity.

Leadership in the group setting is determined by:

- Agency requirements of the worker and group
- Group purpose
- Individual and group needs
- Personality and world view of the worker
- Role of the worker in the group

What distinguishes the leader is the authority given or ascribed to him to influence the group in certain ways, to achieve agreed goals. The employing or funding agency delegates authority to the leader to act on its behalf with a particular group of people. It substantiates this delegated authority with resource, time, and money and in return expects him to behave in certain ways. The group members invest the leader with authority by virtue of his position, skill, or expert knowledge and expect him to be able to move the group to perform the tasks it was called together to do. Whether the leader likes it or not he is required by his agency and perceived by his group to be a person who has authority and power to reward, induce, be an 'expert', be a model, inform, and empower (see page 106).

The first step in working with a group or in preparation for such work is full acceptance by the worker of the fact of his authority to influence and intervene in group experience. There should be no attempt to deny or fudge this. The group worker must claim his authority! Unfortunately many workers have not resolved their own feelings and attitudes to authority and send out conflicting or ambivalent messages about themselves as leaders. The result is to confuse group members, generate insecurity, suspicion, and fear that the worker cannot be relied on in a crisis.

Reluctance or refusal by the group worker to provide leadership to act on his authority can be very damaging at critical stages of transition when the group rightfully look to the worker for guidance, reassurance, and structure. Very often when looking back at why a particular group came to be a conflictual or apathetic experience for people, I have found that the roots lie in the vacuum created by a group worker not facing up to the responsibility and obligations of his authority and failing to provide the group with leadership when it needs boundary and direction.

To determine the nature of his authority base the worker needs to be clear about the requirements and expectations the agency has of him:

- What goals does the agency have for this group?
- What roles and tasks is the worker required to perform with this group?
- What accountability is required of the worker and to whom? (see page 42)
- Are these expectations and requirements compatible with the group goals?

The worker also needs to accept that group members have a right to expect from him:

- Consistency, fairness, honesty
- Recognition of worth, respect, and consideration
- That the worker develops and creates new experiences
- Structure, direction, boundary
- Protection of standards, norms, and values
- Feedback, advice, suggestion
- An increasing and proportionate role in making decisions
- That he act as a model of legitimate and compassionate authority

---

The next step is for the worker to select a model of groupwork which will guide his thinking and understanding of group behaviour, offer suggestions as to leadership style, interventions, and programme. Selection of a groupwork model should be related to the goals of the group, member needs, and the worker's personality and world view. At this stage it is then possible to begin to determine a style of leadership which will accommodate member needs, group goals, and the worker's personal and theoretical perspectives.

We can identify four broad styles of leadership:[1]

- *Directive:* Leader assumes major responsibilities for organizing, convening, guiding, identifying tasks, maintaining flow of ideas and emotions.
- *Permissive:* Leader is non-directive and assumes that if purpose is clear and acceptable, group members can accomplish their goals. The leader does not abdicate his authority but tries to allow the group to determine its own behaviour incentives and strategy.
- *Facilitating:* Leader sees himself as a member of the group but with expertise, role, and function which is different from other members. He places major responsibilities for group process and task accomplishment on the group and its members and tries to be supportive, encouraging, and involved.
- *Flexible:* Leader adapts his position and behaviour in response to his assessment of group functioning, needs of members, and the task and will take up any of the other three leadership styles if it appears appropriate to do so.

In some situations an exclusive or predominant style of leadership may be indicated; disturbed children may require the structure and containment of the more directive stance; a facilitative style of leadership would suit a therapeutic group whereas a community group would benefit from the permissive approach. The style of leadership should be flexible and tailored to the needs and functioning of the individual and the group. For further discussion on this see Chapters 4–7.

Co-leading

The issues of co-leading with more than one worker should be considered carefully in the planning stage. Many group workers start their career co-leading with at least one other worker – very often from a different agency! I have found that lack of preparation and consideration of the nature of the co-leading relationship is a major source of distortion and containment of the group process. My own position is that joint or co-leading is a very sophisticated way of working and not one that I would recommend to the beginner.

For co-leading to be a productive and creative experience:

- Each worker needs to be aware of the contribution of the other, value this, and believe in it.
- Each worker needs to be very clear about his own role and contribution.
- All workers should be clear and in agreement about the purpose of the group.
- All workers should be prepared to fully discuss the conflicts, tensions, and feelings aroused in them by joint work and group experience.
- All workers should be willing to permit and invite differences in perception, style, and approach as long as there is agreement about purpose.
- All workers need to collaborate, share, trust, talk to each other, in and out of the group. The ability of the group to share, deal with conflict and interpersonal issues is directly related to how effective co-leaders are at this.

I often find two extremes in co-leading. On one hand there are the co-leaders who are resentful and jealous of each other. One may feel left out or that his partner is more popular, or does the more glamorous work. Differences in attitude particularly in the sensitive areas of discipline and control can create conflict which is amplified and exacerbated by the presence of group members. The group is quick to spot the presence of latent or explicit conflict, split the workers, and play one off against the other.

On the other hand there are co-leaders who believe it is important to present a united front at all times, irrespective of whatever division there may be in the team. Sometimes this is due to a fear or avoidance of conflict, sometimes to a belief that leader disagreement will have a damaging effect on the group. Both positions are unhealthy.

It is absolutely essential for co-leaders to talk to each other, all the time, in and out of the group, about their perceptions, insights, feelings if they are to exploit co-leading to the full. Reasons put forward in the literature for using co-leaders include the advantages of support, sharing, feedback on each other's performance, time to observe more closely, modelling co-operative leadership, and so on. For me, the real advantage of co-leading is in the willingness of the leaders to exploit and explore their differences in perception of the group experience for the benefit of the individuals and the group.

Differences in perception and response, even lack of agreement, if handled creatively can be an exciting and enhancing experience for group members providing more information, contrasts, and alternatives, offering opportunities for giving opinions, sharing, taking stands, assessment, consideration, and decision-making. In certain situations lack of agreement between leaders may be inevitable. If the relationship is to work the leaders must be able to publicly permit and allow the other's understanding of the situation and value it as a contribution in its own right to the total experience. When this occurs there need be no conflict or necessity to force one viewpoint on the other. Each leader builds on the experience of the other to help the group and its members. Ability to tolerate differing perspectives creates the possibility of synthesis and a new understanding of any and every situation.

Accountability

Much of this will have been worked out when the leader examines the requirements of the agency around the group. Some of the important issues to be clarified here are:

- To whom is the worker accountable?
- Who will guide, monitor, or supervise the worker's practice?
- Who needs to be informed about what is going on in the group?
- How much do they need to know?
- What kind of recording is required?
- Where will it be kept and who will have access to it?

It is important to have clear and explicit agreements or contracts governing these issues, particularly in the sensitive areas relating to communication with colleagues and other agencies interested in the group.

Presenting the group

There are two aspects to presenting the group:

- Presentation of the group to agency for validation, acceptance, permission to proceed, and release of resource.
- Presentation of the group to potential members.

The group should be presented to the agency in planned form. It should consist of a clear, simple, well written proposal containing your thoughts, intentions, and requirements in these areas:

- Background history to proposal.
- Definition of problems to be tackled.
- Purpose, goals, and objectives for the group:
  1 Agency perception;
  2 Member perception.
- Role of worker/s.
- Proposed methodology and programme details.
- Expenditure, resource, transport, equipment required.
- Size of membership, time, date, venue, duration of group, length and frequency of session.
- How you intend to evaluate and assess the value of the group (see page 294).
- Relationships with colleagues or other parties.
- Try to anticipate any possible difficulties that may arise.

Evaluation

An important area to cover in your presentation concerns how you intend to assess and evaluate the success, or otherwise, of the group.[2]
   Try to be clear about your reasons for evaluation:

- To improve the overall functioning of the group.
- To determine if objectives and goals have been achieved.
- To assess whether the group is tackling priority needs and has relevant goals.

- To ensure the group is using resources effectively or identify necessary skills and facilities.
- To improve workers' practice.
- To provide material for supervision.
- To influence policy making.
- To validate the group and ensure its survival and funding.

Consider whether you intend to evaluate:

- *Outcomes:* The extent to which the group achieved its goals in producing change in the targets of intervention.
- *Service delivery:* The types of service offered, their relevance, quality, acceptance, characteristics.
- *Structure and process of the group:* What actually occurred in the group, the quality of work, how it was organized, how resources were used.

Some of the issues you need to think about and a guide to evaluate them are contained in Chapter 13. I raise the subject of evaluation here to remind you that even at the planning stage you should be considering how you intend to assess the effectiveness of the group. The clearer and more specific you are now about what you intend to assess, the easier will be your evaluation at the end of the group. Agencies like to have value for money and indicating to your agency that you fully intend to assess the worth of the group can create a lot of sympathy and goodwill for your proposal.

Presenting the group to potential members

Having presented the group proposal to your agency and obtained approval to start the group, the next step is to meet with potential group members. When I am forming a group I try as far as possible to meet with prospective members before the first session. Referrals will often indicate that a particular person will make a suitable candidate for the group but meeting with them shows that they are patently not suitable for the group: they thought the group was something different; they are only proposing to attend to please the referring agent; or that they are only mildly interested in the group. Without pre-group interviews people can come along to the first two or three sessions in a frame of mind that is unsettling for the group and can be damaging.

I have a number of objectives for the pre-group interview:

To introduce myself (group leader), explain my role in the group, and get a sense of who the prospective member is. While this will not determine the person's behaviour in the group, after interviewing several prospective members I have an impression of how people will get on with each other and have some ideas about what I need to do in the first session with this particular group.

To provide information about the group and its objectives. I try to be very clear about how I see the group and what it is about. It sometimes happens that at this early stage the prospective member can decide that the group is not for them or not what they thought it was. Usually people want to know what we will actually do in the group and seek information about the other members, who they are, what they will be like, will they accept the new member, etc.

To relate the group objectives to the prospective member's perception of need. Without each member being motivated to attend and committed to the group objectives, the group will not work. So it is important to help the prospective member examine his reasons for wanting to join and determine the relevance of the group to his needs. This is a crucial stage because it is easy for the worker to get into 'selling' the group in order to make up the numbers, and not be rigorous about matching member need to group goals. Some prospects can feel intimidated by the worker and against their inclinations may go along with his enthusiasm and conviction. The worker also has to guard against potential members creating unrealistic expectations about the group; there are people who expect immediate 'cures' or deep, intimate relationships by the end of the first session. It is important to short-circuit this by helping the prospect identify specific features or themes in his life which can be worked on in the group, rather than permit global aspirations or expectations. It is easier to use the group, 'to obtain feedback on interpersonal behaviour', than it is to 'use the group to become a happier person'.

Negotiate an individual contract with the prospect. By contract I mean a clear agreement between the prospect and the worker about:

- The purposes and objectives of the group
- The tasks to be undertaken by the prospect in the group
- The prospect's expectations of the worker and the group
- The worker's expectations of the prospect
- The prospect's willingness to attend the group

The particular clauses in the contract are determined very much by the prospective member's acceptance of the legitimacy and relevance of the group for him. One prospect may wish to attend the group for a few sessions to see if it is appropriate for him, so a 'try it and see' clause is more important to him than working out specific tasks to be undertaken in the group. Another prospect may be very willing to accept the group and more energy will go into how he can use the group to achieve certain desired goals.

By making an individual contract with the prospect before the group starts I try to:

- Motivate, engage, and encourage the prospect
- Define what it is that he wants in the group
- Clarify expectations about what is possible, what is not, what is required, what is not
- Emphasize that the prospect is responsible for his use of the group experience
- Show the prospect that he has rights and will not be used against his will
- Demonstrate that the group is designed to be a caring, and compassionate experience

The individual contract will be augmented in the first session by a group contract, made with the other members, but since the prospect only has a contract at this stage with the group worker, it is important to make these agreements as a way of substantiating the idea of the group and engaging the potential member. Individual contracts can be written or verbal; the clauses relating to members' needs and goals can be renegotiated throughout the group experience. Here is a short example of some of the clauses governing expectations that worker and member may have of each other and which can be included in the contract either at pre-group or first session stage.

Our expectations of each other

What you can expect of me	What I expect of you
1 To make available my skills, knowledge and concern to help you make best use of this situation.	1 To help me creat a situation where you can develop, learn, and grow. This means you choose to use me and others appropriately.
2 To be as honest in everything I do with you as I can. I will take risks with you and others in saying what I really think and feel.	2 To be as honest in your dealings with me as you can, take appropriate risks with your thoughts and feelings.
3 To be accepting and supportive of you and ready to clear the air through discussion with you.	3 To take responsibility for your self, your being here, your growth and learning.
4 To allow and assist you to develop your own potential, satisfy your needs for growth and esteem.	4 To be accepting and supportive towards me and the others and ready to clear the air when necessary. Our growth is your growth.

Perhaps you would like to delete some of the clauses and add others of your own.

1 —————————————— 2 ——————————————

John Hodge suggests that an important part of the pre-group interview is to *anticipate the fears and anxieties that the prospect may have* about the group experience and work out ways of acknowledging or resolving these.[3] He suggests that potential members may:

- Wonder what a short-term group can achieve when a problem has existed for years.
- Be fearful that group discussion will undermine their method of coping with problems.
- Be anxious that sessions will be depressing or morbid.
- Worry that sessions will activate feelings and memories they would rather leave undisturbed.
- Be concerned that they will be exposed or may have to give more than they wish.

I find that by bringing these fears and anxieties out into daylight, I give the prospective members permission to have them, can identify potential obstacles to the prospect's participation in the group, and can begin to dispel the more groundless of them. Acknowledgement of the validity of some of these fears, common sense, and compassion, as well as emphasizing the prospect's own power through the contract, all helps to reassure people who have not been a member of a formal group before and who are worried about what they may be letting themselves in for.

My final objective is to *prepare potential members for meeting with the others* in the first session. Typically the prospective member is anxious about speaking in public, revealing his needs or problems, his fears and fantasies about the other members, and generally wonders what it will be like. Explaining the intended format of the first session and reassuring the potential member that everyone else will feel the same as he does can be very comforting. In extreme cases of anxiety I may ask the group member to close his eyes and visually rehearse the whole experience of the first session, preparing him mentally for it and desensitizing the situation of its fear. It is also important to arrange details about transport, time, date, and venue of group sessions as this can be easily forgotten.

The first session

The first session and indeed the early phase of any group is a crucial time for individual members and is critical in determining how subsequent patterns of interaction and communication unfold within the group. Each individual brings to the group his life experience of membership in previous groups and relationships established at earlier stages of his existence.

These experiences will colour his perceptions of and reactions to other group members and the worker. How each member of the group initially presents himself, communicates, behaves, and interacts with the others has enormous repercussions for how the other members will react to him, then and subsequently. Initial impressions can determine how much freedom within the group individuals have to experiment with different aspects of self. Often in the opening sessions group members can become stereotyped and trapped in roles and behaviours that are difficult if not impossible to escape later. For these reasons, it is vital to consider the importance of the first session for individual and group behaviour.

Importance of the first session

- First experience of the group.
- First contact with other members in group context.
- First contact with worker in group context.
- First opportunity to reveal self, behaviour, attitudes, etc.
- First opportunity to hurt or be hurt.
- First opportunity to enjoy the group.
- First opportunity for worker to establish climate, and engage members in work.

With a little reflection, you can extend this list. The important point to grasp is that the *first session is the moment of social and psychological birth for the group*. It is the beginning of familiarization, association, and commitment by individuals to the group life.

Role of the worker in first session

How each individual manages his entry to the group and is facilitated by the other members is crucial if the group is to be seen as a place where persons are valued, and are worthwhile. Central to the whole process at this stage is the worker and his activity in the first session can go a long way towards inhibiting or facilitating group experience. I believe the group worker should try to convey three simple messages to the group in this first session:

The three Cs

Competency: The worker should know what he is doing, be sure about group objectives, his authority, have planned the session thoroughly, and be able to convey to group members that he can be relied on. This does not mean that the worker should cover up his own tension or hide his own natural anxiety. I will share my feelings of tension with the group if it is appropriate, but I am very careful to demonstrate that I am not overwhelmed or incapacitated by them, and that I am competent to work with the group. In this way I normalize feelings of anxiety and act as a role model by showing that I have the power to determine my response to a situation.

Compassion: It is important for the worker to display consideration, concern, care, and compassion for members from the start as a way of setting the tone for group interaction, and helping people feel safe and included. This does not mean that the worker engages in unctuous protestations of care to a group of people he barely knows. Compassion can be easily demonstrated by ensuring that everyone knows and agrees with what is going on, breaking things down and waiting for slower or more defensive members, clearing expectations, making contracts with members, and generally showing that you want to understand and be involved with each member.

Commitment: The worker should display a commitment to and belief in the efficacy and power of the group. Schwarz talks about the worker sharing, 'his own vision of the work' with group members and this is essential at the beginning of the group when members cannot be expected to have a sense of community or even understanding of the power and value of the group experience.[4] If you do not believe in what you are doing or have reservations, you cannot expect members to believe in the group and they will very quickly discern your ambivalence. This applies particularly to those situations where you are thinking of using 'trust games', ice-breakers, and warm-ups (see page 94). Frequently I find group workers using trust games and exercises with people in a group when they readily admit they do not themselves like to be in groups where they are used. Trust games are okay for clients but not for workers! This sort of double standard suggests to me a contempt and lack of understanding of the nature of working with people in group situations. As a basic rule of thumb you should endeavour never to try anything in a group that you are not committed to or believe sincerely to be valuable. And never take a group or its members into any experience you would not be prepared to go into yourself.

Some tips for the first session

Try to sit with people in the group.

Use first names if possible: Use a person's name each time you speak to them. Don't be afraid to ask if you forget. Names are so important as a way of drawing people into the session.

Try to link people together: If a member makes a point, try to link him with those others in the group who feel or think similarly. You are a *weaver* in this first session, trying to intermesh and link people together. Look for the common ground and shared experience between people. Look for themes and patterns that you can reflect. One of the notions I bring into this first session is the idea that we *build on* and add to each other's contributions in order to get a fuller picture. So I'll say things like, 'let's see if we can build on what Mary is saying', or 'let's add to John's point'. The idea here is of the different parts coming together to form a higher-level whole. Each part has an important contribution to make and initially the worker must facilitate the synthesis of the parts.

Expect to be understood: I go into the group clearly expecting to be understood. I also expect members to signal that they don't understand me or each other. To do this I continually ask, 'does this make sense to you?, what is this like for you?' By drawing attention in this way to the need for clarity and comprehension I find that I can encourage more risk-taking, more inquiry, and that members soon learn to feel more confident about stopping the content to share confusion or look for help. I am also clearly stating to the group that I expect them to talk to me in a two-way fashion. I expect group members to reply, question, give their own opinions.

Use plain language and keep your sentences short: Talk to the group members as if you were talking to a friend. Avoid jargon and long-winded descriptions and monologues. Speak simply and briefly and expect a response.

Make your voice, tone, body communicate warmth and interest: Be aware of what you are communicating by your posture, gestures, facial expression. Arms hugging your tummy or your hand around your throat communicate tension and give the lie to your words of calm. Adopt an open, relaxed posture which is comfortable and conveys warmth and attention.

Try to find out what people expect of you, the group, and each other: This is called 'clearing expectations' and is something I believe is essential if you are going to be sensitive to needs and wants of members. Shortly after introductions I build in a space where group members and I can share and discuss our expectations and begin to agree what is realistic, possible, and desirable.

Make a contract with your group and keep it simple: A contract is important for group members. It outlines the rights and responsibilities of worker and member and gives a mark against which all behaviour in the group can be measured and valued (see page 99). Conditions of the contract will vary according to the group but generally you should include clauses about:

- Members' choice to be in the group.
- Confidentiality – what can and cannot be taken out of the group.
- Purposes, objectives of group.
- Time-keeping, breaks, starting times.
- Participation.

We can summarize the role of the worker in the first session:

- To introduce members to each other, the group worker himself, and the group.
- To provide information on group objectives and operation.
- To check expectations and perceptions of group by members.
- To negotiate a contract with members in terms of worker's and members' roles, expectations of each other, purpose of group, etc.
- To minimize frustration and reduce competition and tension.
- To ensure fast satisfaction and success in activity and relationships.
- To facilitate and promote flow of communication between members.
- To invite trust in worker, members, group.
- To encourage exploration.
- To establish the psychological climate of the group and begin to teach the language and procedures for work.
- To engage members in work.

Typical behaviour in the first session

Most groups start cold, shy, and awkward. They most likely do not know each other or the worker and are unsure how to behave. This may be expressed in the following behaviour: milling around; tension due to unfamiliarity; over-dependence on leader; avoidance of each other; silence; superficiality; talking too much; ambivalence and vacillation, etc. (see page 89).

It is essential for the worker to allow what is happening in the group to happen and to help members see group experience as natural, normal, and workable. Thus the worker might decide to reflect what is happening to the group and ask for comment from members. He may point out that it is natural for people meeting for the first time to feel shy and awkward. In this way the worker removes the need for group members to defend and maintain their positions. He accepts the normality of their feeling and draws attention to how members have power to select and determine their responses to situations.

Another way of dealing with the emotional content of the first session is to encourage group members to think about and discuss other first-time experiences, job interviews, what it felt like first day at a new school or job, moving to live in a new neighbourhood, making new friends, and joining new groups.

How to plan the first session

Clarify

- What are your reasons for working with this group?
- What are you expected to do?
- What sort of group is it?
- What is the purpose of the group?
- What are your objectives for the first session?

Consider

- What do you know about the members? Their needs, interests backgrounds, age, sex, size of group.
- How much experience or knowledge do they have about purpose of group or subject of the first session?
- What do they expect of you?

- Try to tune in and anticipate how they may be feeling.
- Spend some time in quiet reflection and meditation to centre yourself.

Context

Try to identify one theme/topic or subject for this session, e.g.:

- Introducing yourself.
- Meeting new people.
- My feelings about beginnings, etc.

This theme is your central thesis for the session, will guide your interventions, enable you to structure feedback, and make sense of group behaviour. The theme gives you a *context* for the session.

Presentation

- Choose methods of presentation which are most appropriate to objectives for the session.
- How do you intend to create the context for this session?
- Design a programme of activity or presentation which is related to abilities and needs of members and session objectives.
- If you decide that you want to reduce tension or facilitate communication think about specific exercises, warm-ups, activities to look at themes like shyness, who I am, meeting and talking to people for the first time.
- Consider how you create consciousness about your theme: debriefs, discussion evaluations, feedback, questionnaires.

Anticipate

Anticipate as many behavioural outcomes as possible but do not be rigid about it.

Consider how to acknowledge and what to do if:

- Members are fearful or unwilling to participate.
- There are long silences.
- Anger or aggression is expressed.
- Members ignore each other and relate only to you.

Ensure

- Co-leaders and special personnel (guest speakers, video operatives, etc.) clearly know what their role is, what is expected of them, and will be there on time.
- Make sure group members know where to come to, what time, what room, are picked up if necessary.

Relax

Enjoy the session. Remember, while it is nice to get everything right in the first session it is not always possible and you will have plenty of opportunities in subsequent sessions to redeem and salvage lost ground. Since most first sessions are carefully planned, they tend to exceed the expectations of workers, so do try to relax!

Some examples of first-session planning

The therapeutic group

Time: Two-and-a-half to three hours.

Setting: A weekly group to explore specific personal problems.

> *Objectives:*
> - To introduce people
> - To provide information about the group
> - To help people say why they have come
> - To build trust and intimacy
> - To promote self-disclosure

Theme: Being together for the first time.

Plan:
- Arrange group seating in small circle to facilitate communication and interaction.
- Provide (optional) soft music to relax, tea, and biscuits.
- Welcome members, start, explain objectives for session. Self introductions (leader directed):

- Who I am.
- How I'm feeling right now.
- Why I'm here tonight.
- My fantasy, expectations, fears about the group. (These statements can be made separately in rounds or all together in one round.)

Leader: Decide whether to evaluate or pass on. If evaluate, decide:

- To give feedback to group on your impressions, feelings
- To give feedback on themes: common problems, shared expectations, mutual fears, fantasies
  or
- To ask group to evaluate self-introductions
  or
- Use themes as basis of discussion, e.g.: being together for the first time; how we are feeling
  or
- Use themes as context for your selection of trust exercises, ice-breakers (see page 94).

Link relevant themes expressed by members to your (leader's) understanding of group purpose.
- Contextualize group (background and history) purposes, aims.
- Indicate how you see the role of leader.
- State your expectations and requirements of members.
- Check and clear expectations and negotiate with members.
- Negotiate a group contract (see page 99). Clauses to include:

- Choice to be here
- Taking responsibility for self
- Attendance
- What I want for myself in this group
- Confidentiality

Share time out between members to focus on:

- What they want from the group
- Why they are here
- What it is like for them to be here for the first time

Do self-disclosure exercises, or a selection of trust exercises, ice-breakers.

Process this work (evaluate it, discuss, share feelings, impressions) in the group with each person or in pairs, threes.

Does anyone need anything at this time?

Review the session: Comments, reflections, feelings

- What I liked about session
- What I didn't like
- How I'm feeling now
- What it was like for me to be here
- Booking time on next session's agenda

Check out (see page 187).

Running a training workshop

Time: Two-and-a-half hours.

Selling: A weekly group to study leadership behaviour in groups.

Objectives:
- To introduce people
- To provide information about group purpose
- To determine people's needs and interests
- To plan a relevant programme
- To develop cohesion and team spirit
- To model leadership behaviour

Theme: Leadership is the process of creating a flexible structure within which people can achieve their goals.

Plan:
- Arrange seating as required. Check equipment.
- Welcome members. Start.
- *General introduction* (leader). Explain: purpose of group, objectives for this session.
- Self introductions:

- Who I am
- Why I am here
- The type of group I lead
- My expectations of the group

- *Negotiate a group contract.* Provide a short summary of need for contract, link this to leadership. Work out clauses.
- *Exercise* to identify member's needs:
- Reflective meditation and writing. Themes to be explored might include:

I   What are my work needs as a group leader?

2   How do I deal with problem behaviours in the group?

3   What are my weaknesses as a leader?

4   What are the qualities and characteristics of the ideal leader?

- Find a partner and share, develop, and expand ideas (fifteen to twenty minutes).
- *Brainstorm* collective needs and interests onto flipchart.
- Categorize areas of need and interest. Prioritize.
- Identify programme units. Discuss and get agreement on an agenda for following sessions.
- Check if group needs a break.
- *Discuss* ways of implementing programme: role play, exercises, case study group discussions. Get agreement on procedures.
- *Select* one theme from checklist for group to work on for

remainder of session, e.g. 'My weakness as a leader' or 'My leadership style'. Brainstorm ideas on it to stimulate group discussion.

or

Split into small groups to explore and discuss a particular feature of the theme. Feedback to larger group.

or

Is theme amenable to role-playing? Set up short scene. Use observers, doubles, and alter-egos to stimulate involvement (see page 206). Finish with group discussion.

- Review session (see page 187)
- Check out.

Making a presentation

Time: Two hours.

Setting: A talk on the relevance of groupwork, to an audience made up of colleagues.

Objectives:
- To stress the universality of group experience
- To identify the positives in group situations
- To point out the relevance of groupwork to a particular clientele
- To allow colleagues to air their views and feelings
- To persuade them groupwork is worth considering

Theme: Group membership is a natural human experience and one that can be used to help people.

Plan:
- Welcome. Start. Indicate your objectives and expectations for session.
- *Brief introduction* to topic covering some of the major issues to be explored.
- *Brainstorm exercise*

---

1 Ask members to identify groups they have belonged to since childhood

2 Pick out four groups. Ask members to identify various benefits of membership

3 Ask members to find a partner. Ask them to assess 'why do people join groups?'. Feedback to group after ten minutes and large group discussion on the three exercises

---

- Leader. Short talk on purposes and aims of groupwork.
- Group *discussion*. Leader: focus discussion on relevance of groupwork to one or two client groups of interest to audience.
- Leader: *summarize themes*, views, feelings of the meeting. Ask for final comments, questions. Make your final statement (see thesis). Thank people for their participation.

Checklist for planning a group

RESEARCH AND JUSTIFY THE NEED FOR GROUPWORK

- How does the demand for group come to your attention? Who makes application, why, for whom, what do they want, what do beneficiaries of the group service actually need?
- What are your reasons for responding to request or requirement to provide a service?
- Gather preliminary information about group (see page 45).
- Decide that groupwork is appropriate for this client or group.
- Identify a general aim.
- Inform colleagues and superiors of your proposal. Request co-operation. Clear lines of communication. Submit a preliminary proposal if possible.
- Gather referrals
- From referrals establish common needs, problems, themes. Begin to identify goals.
- Check goals are consistent with objectives of employing or funding agency. Identify contribution of group to agency service delivery.
- If considering inter-agency work establish each agency objectives, areas of work. Anticipate grey areas or possible difficulties.

ATTENDING TO MEMBERSHIP

- Decide to select, recruit (page 22), work with existing group membership.
- If select:

> - Decide what information you want
> - Gather referrals
> - Assess referrals on descriptive and behavioural attributes (see page 23), common themes, motivation to work

- If recruit:

> - Decide group purpose and goals
> - Advertise – posters, press, word of mouth, clinics, youth clubs, community centres

- If working with existing group membership:

> - Consider what you know of their needs, interests, age, sex, backgrounds
> - Knowledge or experience of group purpose/subject

- Decide on size, frequency, and number of meetings, open or closed groups, duration, length of session.

PROGRAMMING THE GROUP

- Decide why you are going to use a programme.
- Consider needs of members, stage of group development.
- Identify clear objectives.
- Consider how to achieve objectives using activity:

- Determine rules, controls, competence, degree of movement, interaction rewards associated with different activities, personal and task requirements of group
- Consider physical limitations of premises, materials, tools required; how much they cost; where you get the money to pay for them
- Design a relevant programme on basis of all these considerations

- Build review slots into programme.

LEADING THE GROUP

- Analyse and investigate authority base of leader.
- Determine goals of agency:

- Required roles and tasks of worker
- Accountability of worker
- Needs of members

- Consider available models of groupwork. Select an appropriate model to guide thinking and intervention.
- Decide on a style of leadership (see page 40).
- Decide how many workers.
- What are their roles, tasks, functions?
- Anticipate differences, conflicts, and ambiguities between workers.
- Identify to whom worker is accountable (see page 42). Supervision, record keeping, confidentiality.

PRESENTING THE GROUP:

- Write up the group in detail (page 43).
- Present and clear proposals with colleagues and superiors.
- Arrange funding, provision of resource, time, etc.
- Work out how you intend to evaluate the group.

- Present the group to prospective members. Pre-group interviews (see page 44).

PLAN THE FIRST SESSION

- Identify objectives for the session.
- Consider members' needs, interests, backgrounds.
- Select one topic as a context for session.
- Design an appropriate programme of activity.
- Check co-workers, resources, equipment, transport, etc.

Chapter 3

An introduction to group dynamics and process

In the Eastern martial art of aikido, the warrior learns 'never to go against the opponent's strength', but rather to blend with and redirect the energy of his attacker.[1] The aikido master knows how to, 'touch softly and gently' in order to use the power already generated by his adversary. In the midst of motion and conflict there is an exact point to apply pressure and a precise intervention that will subdue the attack. In contrast to this 'way of gentle harmony', the Western disciplines of boxing and wrestling are characterized by collision and force overwhelming force.

The aikido master is a metaphor for the effective group worker who rather than fight or wrestle knows how to be in harmony with his group. He can utilize the pressure points and redirect and employ collective energy and power to take the simplest path towards the desired goal. The simplest path is revealed by awareness and understanding of the meaning of individual and group needs, behaviour, and interaction. Unless he is attentive to and knowledgeable about what is happening inside the system in which he operates an effective group worker cannot adequately determine what is the most appropriate way to intervene or respond.

Unfortunately the study of group dynamics and processes can, at the beginning, be very off-putting and intimidating to the group worker. There are three main problems.

- *Mystique:* At first sight there seems to be so much to assimilate and digest. This is not helped by the impenetrability of much of the language of group dynamics and the reverential attitude of some group workers and the intellectual snobbery of others.
- *Problems of recognition:* Very often the clearly delineated models of group process and development do not match the

confusion of the worker's experience, resulting in frustration, disappointment, and a sense of inadequacy.

- *Problems of application:* Even where certain processes can be identified and recognized many workers are unsure of how to use them in order to create particular effects. In this chapter we will look in detail at how to use group processes to facilitate experience. For now it is enough to clearly and simply identify and present the essential pressure points or group processes which will inform the worker's actions and interventions, and suggest that they are natural and organic events which occur wherever groups of people meet and interact.

Some basic features of group life

Needs and wants of members

A group comes into being to satisfy the needs and wants of its members and unless compelled to do so members will only attend if their needs and expectations are met. In order to understand the behaviour of a group in various circumstances it is important to have firstly a picture of the needs of individuals, and secondly knowledge of how group membership serves each individual. Abraham Maslow offers us an insight into people's needs which we can present as in Figure 3.1.[2]

Maslow suggests that the basic needs for survival and safety have to be met and satisfied if an individual is to progress to the next level of need. Only an unsatisfied need can motivate behaviour and the need which is dominant in an individual is the prime motivator. People deprived of the basic needs abandon higher needs in order to satisfy the lower. If a man's head is held under water for a time he forgets about aesthetic values, social needs, and prestige. He devotes his energy to getting air. Having achieved this he may then move up the scale and feel outraged at this attack on his dignity and act to express this.

The implications of this work are very important for the groupworker:

- Behaviour in the group can be construed as the interplay of one or more member's identification with certain needs.
- Recognition of the need motivating behaviour can indicate the appropriate type of intervention (see page 34).

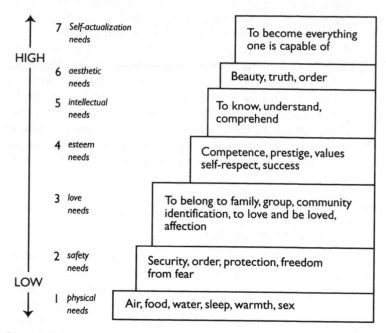

Figure 3.1 Diagram of needs hierarchy

- Recognition of needs is important if you are to successfully develop motivation (see page 205).
- Programme planning must be based on the needs of individuals and the group if it is to be relevant and satisfying. See Chapter 1.

Needs determine goals

No matter how *similar* or *disparate* the needs of individual members, there must be agreement on the *goals* they will strive for while they are in association if the group is to survive and be effective. As the group develops, it continuously works on two levels at once: towards the achievement of group goals and towards the satisfaction of individual member's goals and motives (see page 71). Sometimes individual goals are not shared with other members and may be at cross purposes with the group goals. These *hidden agendas* can be very destructive to the effectiveness of the group and are often the source of conflict in the group. It is important to look for hidden agendas that may be present in the group and encourage their surfacing if appropriate.

Member's commitment to group goals is influenced by:

- How attractive the goal is.
- How realistic it is.
- How challenging and stimulating it is.
- How much satisfaction it represents.

A *goal structure* develops in groups, which indicates the quality of interaction among members. A co-operative goal structure develops when the individual goals of members are visible and similar, e.g. if a member of a quiz team answers correctly, all team members benefit. A competitive goal structure emerges where the individual goals of members are hidden or seen as different or opposed, e.g. in an adolescent group if one member wins the swimming competition, all the other members lose. Some of the effects of co-operation and competition on groups are identified below.

Co-operation	Competition
• Promotes helping, sharing trust	• Decreases helping, sharing trust
• Promotes effective communication	• Makes for ineffective and incomplete communication
• Promotes group cohesion	• Reduces group cohesion, encourages splitting and sub-groups
• Encourages creativity and permits divergence	• Decreases creativity
• Develops interaction and acquisition of skill communication	• Promotes personal skill acquisition at expense of group interaction
• Promotes positive self-attitudes	• Develops loser's and winner's mentality, hostility, distrust, and suspicion

For suggestions on how to develop a co-operative goal structure see page 18.

Goals lead to values

In the course of interacting with each other to achieve personal and group goals members develop a *value system* which refers to beliefs about which objects and behaviours are good and bad, desirable and undesirable. In a therapeutic group whose goal is relief of personal distress, values will emerge which will include an emphasis on honesty, trust, confidentiality, caring, and respect. In an activity group values might include fair play, team spirit, commitment, and sacrifice. The values of a group reflect its goals and purposes, and play an important and often decisive part in determining individual behaviour.

Values make rules

In order to ensure that members behave in accordance with agreed group values and goals, certain rules or *norms* are established which prescribe those actions in particular circumstances which are correct and proper, and those behaviours which are improper. Norms are values expressed in behavioural terms. The acceptance of norms by members depends upon their appropriateness to individual and group concerns, the cohesiveness of the group, and the nature of norm enforcement.

Norms are enforced by *sanctions* which will require or persuade individuals to *conform* to group values and beliefs. These sanctions will punish members who fail to conform to group norms or reward them if they do so adequately. In our example of the therapeutic group, violation of the norm of confidentiality might be met with demands for removal or 'expulsion' of the offender. In the activity group conspicuous adherence to the norm of fair play could result in an individual being rewarded with the rank of team captain or arbiter of standards.

The group's impulse to create norms and behavioural controls can be of great benefit to you when working with the group. Most beginning workers seek to establish *personal control* over the group fairly early on. They fail to realize that the most effective means of control within any group is that based on establishing norms of behaviour which are acceptable to all and identifying and using those norms which already exist. By trying to develop and make satisfying and rewarding existent norms, you will find that you are likely to be more successful than trying to control the group externally (see page 95).

Rules lead to roles

The emergence of group goals, values, and norms requires the members to behave in a co-ordinated and standardized way if group discussion, planning together, or participating in a particular activity is to occur. However, even within the standardized action patterns of a group, a wide range of behaviours and operations may be necessary in order to achieve the task or goal. Group discussion for example can be broken down into a set of sub-tasks: someone has to select or offer a theme, other members are required to give opinions, listen, share views, suggest alternatives, and engage in the repertoire of behaviours which will facilitate group discussion.

A division of labour begins to develop with individuals allocated certain tasks and functions. Over time these become institutionalized as *roles* in the group. The term 'role' derives from the theatre where an actor may perform in the role of Hamlet or Basil Fawlty or a king. A role is a series of actions which guide and determine our behaviour according to what is expected of us in a certain situation. Roles generate the consistency and predictability of behaviour which we have seen is so important in group life and create expectations about how members will behave in relation to each other and the group goals.

Throughout life we perform many roles as son/daughter, friend/lover, employer/employee and so in groups we engage in role behaviour as member, follower, and leader amongst others. This information is vital to the group worker because now any behaviour of any member can be questioned: 'What role do these actions represent and is it appropriate?' Let's see how this can be developed.

All roles are functional in that they serve individual and group interests in some way. But problems can arise.

People are induced to occupy certain roles because of group pressure to *conform* to expectations and norms. Sometimes group pressure to conform can be very intense and individuals outwardly conform to the norm out of fear while inwardly disagreeing. This can have disastrous results for the group, ranging from apathy and impotence to sabotage and acts of defiance.

Each role carries a measurement of worth. Some roles are more valuable and sought after by members than others, because they have more *status*. The role of leader usually carries high status while the *scapegoat* denotes low status and may be ascribed to a member of the group who is unpopular or disagreeable. Role status can be used as a reward or punishment and leads to the development of a social structure, usually hierarchical, which can stratify members, reduce mobility and cohesion, and create sub-groups.

Because of a lack of flexibility and role fluidity individuals can come to be *locked* into a role. *Role lock* limits the opportunities and options in interpersonal relationships and creates rigid and stereotyped behaviour. This fixed position may be chosen by an individual or ascribed to him but either way is used to prevent change, remain static, and avoid responsibility.

Role conflict can develop because:

- Members are obliged to occupy roles which carry expectations and instructions for behaviour which are incompatible or disagreeable to them.
- Two people may make opposing or conflicting demands on the role holder. This happens frequently in groups where the leader wants a member to behave in a way which will alienate him from his peers, e.g., 'tell me who stole the biscuits!'
- Often we fill so many different roles in rapid succession and the demands of one may conflict with the demands of another, e.g. my role as group leader conflicts with my role as husband when I have to work yet another weekend group.

Group performance and effectiveness can be seen as the interplay of three main sets of needs and behaviours each of which gives rise to a series of formal and informal roles (Figure 3.2). These functional roles of group members were first described by Benne and Sheats in 1948 and have been used continuously since then.[3,4,5]

The first circle refers to those needs, behaviours, and roles that are required to help the group achieve its goals. The second circle encompasses those behaviours and roles that help the group look after its emotional and interpersonal well-being. The third circle is concerned with the purely personal motives of each individual. The circles overlap because some behaviours are task- and maintenance-oriented at the same time, and because all task and maintenance behaviours are mediated by personal motivations which can result in positive or anti-group behaviours and roles. We can begin to

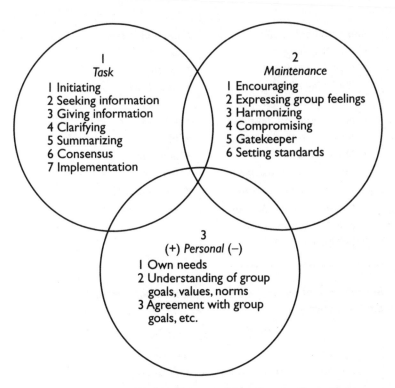

Figure 3.2 Task, maintenance, and personal functions in the group

identify members' behaviours, and the roles with which they are associated over time, in terms of whether they impede or facilitate the group.

Behaviours and roles related to members' needs rather than the task

In each of the behaviours and roles listed on page 72, personal need is taking precedence over collective need. A group member may not be able to adequately listen to others because he desperately needs listening to himself. Try to identify the need motivating behaviour and role in order to make your intervention and responses more relevant and sensitive (see page 66).

Anti-group behaviours	Anti-group roles
• Not listening	• Blocker
• Cutting people short	• Avoider
• Deflating people	• Saboteur
• Picking on people	• Critic
• Nit-picking on details	• Dominator
• Refusing to yield	• Martyr
• Messing about	• Scapegoat
• Inappropriate joking, sarcasm, black humour	• Isolate
• Inappropriate aggression, anger, arguments	• Double/cynic
• Self-pity	• Persecutor

Behaviours and roles aimed at helping members interact more effectively

Pro-group behaviours	Pro-group roles
• Involving other members	• Encourager
• Reconciling disagreements	• Harmonizer
• Praising people	• Gatekeeper
• Communicating	• Standard setter
• Relieving tension	• Mediator
• Co-operating	
• Encouraging and exhorting people	
• Listening to others	

Behaviours and roles focused on accomplishing the group goal

In the behaviours and roles on page 73 the group member is not feeling deprived or deficient but is focusing on other people or the task from his own needs to contribute to the group, be a part of what is happening, join in. Your response in this situation might be more to permit this, facilitate, and acknowledge individual efforts.

Pro-group behaviours	Pro-group roles
• Starting things • Sharing information and resources • Organizing activity and members • Giving opinions • Asking opinions • Elaborating and explaining • Looking for agreement • Summarizing	• Initiator • Orienter • Co-ordinator • Evaluator

Questions to ask yourself about role-behaviour in the group

• Is this behaviour recurrent enough to be called a role?
• How would I describe this role? What is this person saying to me and the group through the role?
• Does the individual seem happy with this role?
• Is he trapped in this role?
• Is he experiencing role conflict?
• What status or position in the group accrues to this person as a result of this role?
• What are the gains and losses to the group of this person conforming in his role?
• What is the individual's perception of his role?
• Is this role related to task, maintenance, or personal needs?
• What does the individual need or want in order to change, develop, be more included in the group?

Group process

These aspects of group culture that we have been looking at are outward manifestations of the group process. Group process is one of the most hallowed dogmas in the modern groupwork liturgy, and to beginners one of the most confusing. We are going to look in detail at what group process is and why it is so important but first it is necessary to distinguish between the content and the process of a group.

- Content refers to the *what* of group experience – what is being talked about, what activity is taking place, what the group members are going to do next.
- Process refers to the *how* of group experience, the *way* in which a group discusses or acts together and is reflected in the quality of group experience.
- Content is the substance of group activity which can be clearly seen on the surface and gives the members a *social* context within which they can interact. It is usually manifest and *seen*.
- In contrast, process is what happens underneath the surface on the psychological level of group operations. It is usually latent and *felt*.

Group process as a frame of reference

From this perspective group process is, 'a frame of reference which limits, focuses and directs the worker's efforts in a group'.[6] It is based on the assumption that group process can be 'controlled and influenced by the worker's actions'. Group process can be defined as changes over time in the internal structure, organizations, and culture of the:

- Whole group
- Part of the group
- Individual member

and expressed

1 *Structurally* in the:
- Effectiveness of communication
- Quality of decision making
- Allocation of roles
- Quality of power and authority in group
- Calibre of group culture, norms, values, goals

2 *Behaviourally* in the:
- Quality of interaction
- Silence, anger, tears, avoidance
- Lateness, absenteeism, getting stuck
- Gesture, posture
- Seating arrangements

3 *Psychologically* in the:
- Degree of trust, cohesion, intimacy
- Extent to which individual feels:
  - Valued
  - Included
  - Able to contribute
  - Defensive versus open
  - Split or integrated

Let me draw attention to a number of important principles in this process approach to working with a group:

- Individual and group experience and interaction *change condition* over time. There is movement, flux, and process. This flux and change is not random or chaotic but is *organic* and natural. There is an ebb and flow, a development and decline that we can call process. It is possible to discern themes and patterns in this movement (see page 79).
- Individual and group experience has distinct *energetic* manifestations:
  - The tension of strangeness and embarrassment.
  - The cold of silence and indifference.
  - The heat and rush of anger.
  - The warmth of companionship and co-operation.

The fact that group experience and interaction can be emotionally and physically felt means we can quite easily develop skills of working with process by becoming more receptive and open to what is occurring.

- Like the aikido master who used the energy and momentum of his adversary's attack to subdue him, the group worker can influence, alter, and control the energy manifested at any stage of the group process. For example, knowing that a group of people are meeting for the first time we can design a programme in the opening sessions which is nurturing and warm and helps people with the business of inclusion (see pages 88–102); or seeing that members keep getting stuck at a particular point we can intervene from a number of angles to help people with the experience (see page 34).

- Individual and group experience and interaction is continuously unfolding in the present tense of group life. Because of the 'nowness' of process every experience is open to change. Attending to individual and group phenomena as they occur right here and now gives members the potential and opportunity to change direction and devise new strategies. Each member can learn to become a participant observer because he is in the events that concern him, and making them happen at the same time that he is watching them. This can be a difficult experience for members at first, and methods for process analysis may have to be built in so that group members come to learn that it can be productive to take time out from *what* is happening to look at *how* it is happening

  For the leader, working with group process can at times be like a canoeist negotiating tumultuous white water rapids – you have to roll under this wave, block that one, switch direction suddenly, be swept along by the river for a time, then head for the bank, swerve, sway, lean, and pray!

Love and will polarities in the group

In the introduction we identified the drive mechanism for movement and growth in groups as deriving from the tension generated between two poles of human psychology – the urge to be attached and the urge to separate. That human experience can be considered as the manifestation of two opposing but complementary polarities requires to be demonstrated and in order to do this we need to examine the quality, nature, and direction of the opposing tendencies. For convenience I shall call the urge to be attached, the love principle and designate the urge to be separate as the will principle.

I do not mean that the love principle is simply a matter of feeling or affect. Assagioli asserts that the varied manifestations of the love principle 'express the law of attraction, of the tendency towards approach, contact, unification and fusion'.[7] Andreas Angyal calls it the 'trend towards homonymy' and describes it as the tendency by which, 'a person seeks union with larger units and wishes to share and participate in something which he regards as being greater than his individual self'.[8] We can state some of its functions and qualities:

Functions	Qualities
• Relating	• Nurturance
• Uniting	• Sensitivity
• Fusing	• Reciprocity
• Connecting	• Identification
• Attachment	• Intimacy
• Possession	• Compassion
• Understanding	• Support

The love principle manifests in human behaviour which is magnetic, connective, and inclusive:

Behaviours	Distortions
• Making friends	• Shyness
• Joining in	• Embarrassment
• Taking sides	• Fear of rejection
• Conversation	• Superficiality
• Sharing	• Silence
• Trusting	• Jealousy
• Co-operating	• Suspicion
• Encouraging	• Hostility

The will principle is characterized by its tendency to separate, initiate, and dominate. Angyal sees the will as an expression of 'autonomy', the capacity of an organism to operate according to its own nature rather than under the control of external forces.[9] Evolution can be understood in terms of this energy, as the graduations from vegetable kingdom to man are characterized by an increasing ability to differentiate and self-determine.

Assagioli states that, 'the most important personal characteristic of the will type is the will to power'.[10] This is expressed in the desire to lead or dominate. Degenerate forms of the will to power result in selfishness, stubbornness, and contempt.

Functions	Qualities
• Separate	• Vision
• Differentiate	• Purpose
• Lead	• Persistence
• Govern	• Independence
• Determine	• Self-reliance
• Action	• Courage
• Judge	• Control
• Complete	• Power

The will principle manifests itself in human behaviour which is separative, exclusive, and concerned with mobilizing power and energy.

Behaviours	Distortions
• Starting things	• Rivalry
• Organizing activity	• Stubbornness
• Leading	• Selfishness
• Sub-grouping	• Powerlessness
• Problem-solving	• Apathy
• Decision-making	• Restlessness
• Concentration	• Violence
• Confrontation	

It should be clear now that psychological and interpersonal life is the consequence and manifestation of the tension generated by love and will polarities in the group. Each individual and the group as a whole has to reconcile these opposites if the experience is to be productive and worthwhile.

Each reconciliation of the opposite is a synthesis of the essential elements in each. Synthesis differentiates new behaviour and experience and produces an upwardly spiralling effect. This makes for an intensification and a refining of the quality of experience at different levels and at different stages in the development of the group. It is through this upwardly spiralling synthesis that the group grows and matures.

Sometimes the process is characterized by a protracted series of conflicts, crises, approaches, and avoidances, as group members oscillate between the two extremes. At other times the process is more harmonious and members are able to synthesize and transmute the polar energies. In the next section we will look at some of the typical patterns in the process and in Chapters 4 to 7 suggest ways in which the worker can work with and facilitate group development.

Patterns and stages in group process

It is apparent that group conditions change over time as a consequence of the energy generated by love and will polarities in the group. Observing and understanding the change in conditions is a basic skill of groupwork practice. By analysing the oscillation in condition and discerning the themes and patterns of interaction, relationship, and behaviour, it is possible to determine what needs prevail in the group at any given time, and permit intervention to emerge out of the particular group situation.

Most writers describe a series of phases or stages in the developmental patterns of the group. Schutz for example has suggested a three-stage scheme of (1) inclusion, (2) control, (3) affection.[11] Tuckman describes four stages in group development: (1) forming, (2) storming, (3) norming, (4) performing.[12] Garland, Jones, and Kolodny insist there are five stages: (1) pre-affiliation, (2) power and control, (3) intimacy, (4) differentiation, and (5) separation.[13] If we ignore the number of stages, what emerges from these writings is a description of the interplay of love and will energies in the group. Although they use different words each writer is clearly talking about the effect of these two principles on group interaction and development.

Tuckman, Garland, and his colleagues in common with many writers assume a linear or sequential progression in group development. As we observed earlier (page 64) this academic and orderly delineation of group process can be alien to the experience of many beginning group workers as they survey the apparent chaos and confusion of their own groups. Groups clearly do not only move sequentially through neat phases, but also move backwards and sideways as well as forwards. Again, each group differs in the amount of time it spends in a particular stage of growth and some groups can get stuck and never progress beyond a certain stage.

The three-stage formulation of Schutz goes some way towards allowing for lateral and retrograde mobility. Schutz hypothesizes three linear phases but he does suggest the notion of circularity and spiralling. In other words a group can reverse and repeat sequences and can move forward by apparently going back through stages and even by going around in circles.

The first stage of group development is, according to Schutz, the *inclusion phase*. Inclusion behaviour refers to the desire to connect to and associate with other people, to want interaction and relationship. This is a period when group members are acclimatizing to the group and becoming familiar with each other though they have not yet formed close ties. There is a lot of restlessness, tension, and mobility. Members are evaluating and probing each other for mutual or complementary interests, exploring possibilities and beginning some preliminary pairing. (For a detailed description of typical behaviours at this stage see page 89.) Tuckman sees orientation, testing, and the establishment of dependancy relationships by group members as the chief characteristic of this phase.

The central issue for members at this stage is to belong to the group or not, to be in or out. Garland and his colleagues highlight the ambivalence experienced by members. They identify two divergent tendencies operating in the individual, 'the tendency to approach and involve himself', and 'the tendency to avoid the situation because of the demands, the frustrations and even the pain which he may anticipate'.[14] As we shall see in Chapter 4 there is a great deal that the worker can do to help members recognize and resolve their inclusion issues and establish a sense of belonging.

Once the problem of inclusion has been satisfactorily resolved, Schutz suggests that *control* issues become prominent. Control behaviour is the independent and assertive activity of group members in the areas of power, authority, status, influence, decision-making, and communication and would be equivalent to our will principle in operation.

Once the group has begun to form it starts to differentiate and develop a social structure. People assume or are ascribed roles and functions, positions and ranks. Cliques form and alliances are made as members jockey for status and power. There are two central issues for members at this stage:

- How much influence can they exercise in the group.
- How much personal autonomy do they have to surrender in order to be part of the group.

Members often compete against the formal authority vested in the group worker. At times this is an attempt to determine how much control they have and how much the worker has over events in the group. At other times the testing of the worker is a boundary-setting exercise, an attempt to determine what is and what is not permissible in the group. Members also conflict with the worker as a way of establishing his competency, ascertaining that he can be depended on, that he can maintain control, and can be trusted.

The struggle between members is, according to Garland and his colleagues, 'an attempt to define and formalize relationships and create a status hierarchy'.[15] Members come to this new group from other settings and have to renegotiate and establish their positions and identities. The discomfort of creating and adjusting to a new social structure can manifest itself in a variety of behaviours such as hostility, scapegoating, withdrawal, sub-grouping, power struggles, and deviance which take members *away* from each other and pit them *against* each other (see page 105).

In my experience this is the phase of group development least understood and most threatening to the beginning group worker. A previously docile or compliant group can suddenly erupt into conflict, bickering, and apparent mutiny. A therapy group may turn on the leader, a work group may split into factions. It is a tempestuous time for worker and group alike as can be seen by Tuckman's description of this phase of development as 'storming'. Hartford calls it a period of 'disintegration followed by rapid termination or reintegration'.[16]

While groups can get stuck in this phase, the flux and dynamism of the turmoil brings with it much potential for reconstituting the group relationships on a higher level of involvement. Confirmation of this, and for the worker – words of comfort – can be found in the I Ching or Chinese Book of Changes which makes change itself the purpose and meaning of life. In a commentary on 'Chen', the Chinese word for 'thunder' (Hexagram 51) the I Ching asserts that 'Thunder indicates success', and goes on to say that, 'it laughs and shouts in fearful glee, yet afterwards everything is in order'.[17] And anticipating Hartford by some 3,500 years in a commentary on 'Huan' meaning 'disintegration' (Hexagram 59) the I Ching states that 'Dispersion leads to accumulation, but this is not something that ordinary people understand'.[18]

In accordance with these laws of transformation the will energies of the group give way and love energies begin to predominate. These love energies operate on a higher level than the love energies of the earlier inclusion stage. Whereas the inclusion stage is about the decision to belong or not, this *affection* stage as Schutz calls it, is about building emotional ties and deciding on the degree of intimacy to be developed with the other group members. Garland and his colleagues in fact call this the stage of *intimacy*. More prosaically, Tuckman calls it *norming* although he emphasizes, 'intimate, personal opinions are expressed'.[19]

In this period the group assumes an importance for members. There is a sense of identity and pulling together. Participation and involvement increase and members are more sensitive to each other. The interpersonal relationships stabilize and it is possible to observe the heightened emotional feeling between pairs of members, triads, and sub-groups. The group is increasingly experienced as a trustworthy supportive environment. This leads to more genuine encounter and interaction.

Tuckman and Garland now see the group move up another level under the influx of more integrative will energies. In what Tuckman calls the *performing* stage the structure of the group has evolved to the point where it is 'supportive of task performance'. Roles have become flexible and functional 'and group energy is channelled into the task'.[20] Garland and his colleagues call this fourth progression, *differentiation*. People begin to acknowledge each other's uniqueness and permit individual differences to emerge. The standards and norms of behaviour are established and increasing reference is made to the internal mores rather than to external values and associations.

Increasing differentiation in the group finds its natural expression in the ultimate *separation* of group members, although Garland and his colleagues see separation as a distinct phase. However, they do agree with Schutz that separation involves 'regression and recapitulation', a spiralling back through earlier phases. Schutz suggests that as groups terminate they deal firstly with the personal feelings of members about closure (affection) then decide to comply or rebel against the leader's wishes (control), before finally discussing the possibilities of continuing the group, assessing the original commitment of members, and preparing for entry into the outside world (inclusion). In Chapter 4 we will come back to explore these patterns in group process in more detail as a way of suggesting how you can co-operate with, influence, and intervene in group process in a relaxed and organic fashion.

Stages theory is a map, not the territory

It is important to recognize that like human fingerprints, no two groups are identical in their development. Every group experience is unique and will not strictly adhere to a neat model of sequential phases. Groups are in motion all the time and there is overlap, spiralling, regression, and continual oscillation between the polarities of love and will in the group. At times both energies are clearly operative in the group, particularly at transition points, and the group has the option of staying put, regressing, or going forward. There is no guarantee that the group will automatically progress and because of this it is essential that the worker is attentive to what is actually happening in the group in terms of members' love and will needs and issues, rather than looking for confirmation of a favourite model.

Many workers in my experience come unstuck, become frustrated, and even doubt their own competence when their groups do not appear to follow the neat schemata outlined in the groupwork texts. It is important to remember that stages theory is only a map. It is *not* the actual territory. The territory must be negotiated as it is being traversed. The map can offer pointers and markers but only if it is intelligently used and not slavishly followed.

Review

- While every group is unique there are certain basic features of culture and structure.
- Behaviour is not random.
- Behaviour is comprehensible.
- Behaviour can be anticipated.
- Behaviour in the group is best understood at the level of group process, rather than solely in terms of individual personality.
- The drive mechanism in group process is the tension generated

by the archetypal urge to attach and its opposite, the urge to separate.

- Group process is organic and displays unfolding themes and patterns of growth and development.
- It is possible to recognize these themes and patterns and influence them.

Chapter 4

Work at the beginning stages of the group: inclusion issues

In the last chapter I said that it was possible for the worker to consciously co-operate with the organic processes of growth and development in the group in order to liberate and utilize its creative energy and resource. A statement like this immediately raises questions about what precisely it is that the group worker co-operates with and how he goes about it.

The answer is quite simple when one remembers that movement and change occur as a consequence of the energy generated by the tension between the love and will polarities which are always present in the group.

However, in the volatile, rowdy, and often apparently chaotic atmosphere of many groups the beginning group worker can find that he lacks the expertise and confidence which would help him understand and feel competent to deal with what is happening. With this thought in mind I have written this chapter to help you recognize what these love and will energies actually look like in the group and how they influence behaviour. I have also included specific instructions on how to use these energies to enhance the process of the group. Before moving to this let me mention three basic principles that will recur.

The group is organic and capable of evolving

What I mean by this is that group experience is an organic and unfolding process in which behaviour is neither random nor illogical but can be discerned as comprehensible themes and patterns of experience and need. The group is not in its essential nature a chaotic, static, or inert phenomenon. Groups are energetically dynamic and tend to develop in an increasingly inclusive and more organized manner.

Behaviour reveals its meaning when seen in context

Following on from this is my belief that observing and understanding these themes and patterns is the first and most basic skill for groupwork practice. You will not know how to respond, how to intervene, or help your group if you cannot see and accurately understand what is happening between people.

How are you to make sense of the events that you are experiencing in a group situation? When two people argue, for example, are they merely expressing differing viewpoints? Do they not like each other? Could it be that they feel unsafe in the group? Do they not understand what they are supposed to do? And how are you to intervene? How can you know what exactly is taking place?

What I am pointing to here is the *meaning* that we attribute to a particular interaction or event; the real nature of what it is that you are looking at, hearing, or attending to. An organism and its actions are not independent of its environment. There is a clear relationship between the whole and its parts and when we blur or avoid this relationship we often cannot see the wood for the trees. Unfortunately many new group workers have a tendency to respond to events in the group at an immediate and surface level, failing or forgetting to see these events in the context of group life. They can experience group behaviour as random, illogical, and meaningless and often find their interventions are uninformed, lacking in precision, and too emotive.

The meaning or nature of an event or interaction can only be fully understood when it is seen against the background or in the context in which it occurs. Nothing exists without a context or ground. Clouds are seen against the background of the sky, waves against the sea, and you are able to recognize these words because they are set against the whiteness of the page. So the meaning of a specific behaviour or interaction in a group should always be seen in the context of that particular stage of group unfolding.

The importance of love and will energies

The third theme which we will explore is concerned with how the leader uses the love and will energies in his own psyche as well as in the group, to relate to members individually and collectively. The point here is that whilst everyone has available to them the love and will energies, men and women are traditionally cast in typical sex roles which tend to overdevelop certain energies and qualities of the self at the expense of underdeveloping others. For example, men are expected to be more concerned with the will and assertion energies in everyday life and women are required to operate more under the influence of the love principle. I am not saying by this that men are unable to be caring or sensitive or that women cannot be assertive or competitive. I am pointing to common attitudes and experiences which I believe have important implications for working with groups. What I am saying is that when working with a group, leaders should be careful not to operate solely out of their usual sex-role identifications or the group will tend to develop in a one-sided way. Following the example of the leader, members may avoid conflict, scorn the expression of feelings, be overly competitive, or uncomfortable with vulnerability.

Irrespective of gender the group worker needs to use both the masculine and feminine energies in the self if the group experience is not to be impoverished. Workers should give careful thought to ways in which they might transcend stereotyped sex roles at important stages in the group life. A male worker could consider how to more consciously use the love energies available to him in order to meet group needs for reassurance, protection, and sympathy. A female worker could consider how to employ her will energies to provide the group with an experience of boundary, consistency, and order.

The importance of the worker being able to use the love and will energies in himself is underscored if we consider the group as a representation of the archetypal family. Irrespective of age or ability and despite the purpose or task for which the group was set up there is a level at which individuals can come into relationship with the leader and the other members as if with the parent and siblings in the archetypal family. This can be readily seen in any group at different stages of its life where individual members act towards each other and particularly the leader in a dependent, aggressive, rebellious, or jealous manner.

On these occasions the worker and his colleagues in the group come to embody for individuals the love and will energies involved in parenting – the mother and father aspects of the archetypal parent. So at different times in the group members will look to the worker for certain parenting responses. As we shall see, in the inclusion period of the group members are dependent and anxious and will look for a nurturing or positive mothering approach from the worker. As the group successfully resolves its ambivalence about inclusion, the mothering side of the worker has to be experienced as negative so that members can separate from him and begin to explore relationships with each other.

There ensues a time of conflict and aggression; of seeking after power and challenging authority. The group now looks to the worker to use the will energies of the archetypal father to model leadership, give structure, and permit appropriate rebellion. In time the group passes through the 'control' stage to the more mature and interdependent relationships of the 'affection' stage of group life. Here members are able to transcend the love and will issues of the two previous stages and relate to the leader and each other in a more adult manner. It is as if members have used the maternal and paternal qualities of the earlier stages to create the atmosphere in which they can now begin to individuate and use the group reciprocally to benefit themselves and each other.

From this brief discussion it is clear that the worker needs to recognize and be able to use both the love and will/assertion energies in himself as well as in the group. A negative and often destructive spiral can easily develop if the worker does not realize what is taking place and makes an inappropriate will or love type intervention. Just as with parents, group members will react against the inappropriate response with all the old stereotyped strategies of childhood.

Inclusion issues

Recognition

Whether the group is a counselling, work, educational, or recreational experience, the first issue that emerges as soon as people come together is about belonging. From the start each individual has to decide to be part of the group or not; to be *in* or *out*. At the same time each individual has to decide his degree of commitment to and inclusion in the group. How much or how little contact, interaction, and communication does he wish to engage in?

At the inclusion stage group members may engage in a wide variety of behaviours as a way of resolving their anxieties and preoccupations. These anxieties result from the conflict and demands of two divergent tendencies operating in the mind of uncertain members. On the one hand the momentum of the love principle generates a concern to attach, belong, relate, connect with other people (see page 76). The impulse to belong is further enhanced by the strength of the individual's desire for *this* group experience; for the gratifications promised in *this* group opportunity. On the other hand the will principle generates an impulse to separate and be independent (see page 78). This is partly because of the demands, frustrations, and anxieties that may be anticipated and is often fuelled by memories and experiences of previous groups (see boxes below and page 90).

These opposing tendencies create tension and ambivalence and cause the potential member to ask himself questions such as:

- What will the other members be like? What will they think of me? Will I fit in? Can I trust them? Will I like them?
- What kind of group is this? Can I get what I need in this group? What do I have to do here? Can I cope in this group? Will it be a good group?
- What is the leader going to be like? Can I trust him? Is he

Moving towards other group members (Love principle)	*Underlying needs and motives*

• Introductions
• Initiating conversations 'cocktail party talk'
  Themes: weather, football, government, people we know
• Sharing of similar/previous experiences
  Establishing mutuality
• Joining in activities
• Exploring/examining environment, equipment
• Sharing space, material, food, equipment, conversation, self
• Establishing rules, procedures
• Humour, joking, teasing
• Depending on the leader
• Beginning relationships
	• To approach, connect, belong, be part of, interact
	• To be protected, feel secure, have order, system, rule
	• To encounter other members, know them, assess them
	• To be regarded as worthwhile, significant, valuable
	• To determine possibilities offered by the group

Moving away from or against other group members (Will principle)	Underlying needs and motives
• Absenteeism • Lateness • Silence • Halting/sporadic conversations • Talking too much/ chattering • Repetitiveness/asking for instructions, information previously given, going over ground again • Superficiality, skimming/ glossing over issues • Preoccupation with tasks, procedures, and rules • Refusing to join in activities, withdrawal, self-sufficiency • Expressions of boredom, contempt, indifference • Hovering, hesitation, fence-sitting, edge of group activity, distancing, suggestions for separative activity, e.g. hide and go seek • Impulsive behaviour, greed, aggression, random activity • Vandalism of furniture, equipment, environment • Exhibitionistic behaviour, attention-seeking, showing off, boasting • Over-dependence on the leader	• Fear of being rejected, attacked, ridiculed, making a mistake • Need to assert self as competent and significant, valuable, worthwhile • Fear of being taken over by group, of being obligated, committed, coerced • Fear of being dependent, needy, vulnerable • Need to avoid close association • Need to defend and maintain a separative self • Unwillingness to trust others • Need to 'wait and see' • Need for order, direction, security, protection, safety

dependable? Will he like me? Whom will he like best? Will he be strict?

Anxiety about these issues is expressed in this opening phase of group life in the form of individual-centred behaviour which satisfies both the love and the will impulses simultaneously, in behaviour which facilitates involvement, exploration, and self-disclosure while at the same time permits some distance and protection from too much encounter too soon.

It is possible to identify some of the more usual patterns of behaviour in the opening sessions of the group. Remember that there is no clear-cut sequence in which one behaviour follows from another! Each group is unique and depending on its goals and the nature and motivations of the people who make it up, one, some, or all of these behaviours may be apparent on different occasions in the beginning.

Mothering: nurturing the group at the inclusion stage

Guiding the group through the inclusion stage demands a great deal of awareness and sensitivity from the worker. The prime requirement is to 'see' behaviour in the opening sessions as the expression of a very natural 'approach-avoid' ambivalence; as the way in which potential members struggle with and reconcile the tensions and implications of beginning group membership.

A perspective like this shapes the way a worker relates to the group. Now, interventions are made not so much to correct or proscribe behaviour, but rather to positively respond to and use the love and will needs being expressed in particular behaviours.

Knowing how people are likely to feel and behave the worker can conduct himself in such a way, and provide a programme which minimizes anxiety and frustration and reinforces the desire of members to join in. Similarly, instead of getting exasperated or feeling inadequate about members' unwillingness to participate in activity, their silence, or superficiality, a worker might decide to go beneath the behaviour to *acknowledge* and *permit* people's fears in new situations. By involving members in discussion about their anxieties and their needs the worker communicates a clear message that it is alright to be anxious and that something can be done about it. The worker also begins to create an environment which values and facilitates awareness and choice rather than compulsive and fear-determined behaviour.

But what precisely, does the worker do at this stage? I would suggest that the worker's operations derive from the fact that the group is a multi-dimensional experience. There are layers or levels of experience mediated by the love–will polarity, which influence and determine individual and group behaviour. These layers or levels of experience can operate simultaneously as well as hierarchically and will usually produce some confusion for members.

There is a *physical* level at which members need and want to interact but may worry perhaps about how touching each other will be construed. People get tired, restless, and want to move. They react to noise, cold, distractions in the environment, the size of the room, and seating arrangements.

At the *feeling level* members can be anxious, fearful, shy, and embarrassed. At other times they may be eager, excited, or impulsive. On an *intellectual level* members usually have questions about the group, its objectives, purposes, methods of working and are curious about each other's background and reasons for being in the group.

The range of behaviours which may manifest on these different levels of group experience suggest four major tasks for the worker at this stage:

- Fostering members' attraction to the group.
- Establishing structure and control.
- Developing trust and cohesion.
- Negotiating agreement on the work of the group.

In practice, I find that these tasks tend not to be very separate and discrete but rather form a continuum of worker activity that is distinctly 'nurturing' in style and effect. When I talk about 'nurturing the group' I mean that I try to nourish and reassure members at the physical, emotional, and intellectual levels of group experience. In other words I attempt to create an atmosphere which is warm, gentle, and friendly, accepting but purposeful, and which inspires trust. A metaphor which I consciously employ here is of the '*worker as group mother*'.

I believe that the opening sequence of the group calls for a gentle, nurturing approach irrespective of the worker's sex, an approach which tends to be associated with females and mother. Earlier I said that the first session was the moment of social and psychological birth (page 49) and so the inclusion stage of group life can be likened to the time of infancy and childhood.

There is a certain level at which, regardless of age, each prospective member relates to the leader and the other group members as might a child. This can be seen in the kind of questions the member brings to the group (see page 89). This does not mean that the individual is childish but rather that the prospective member comes to group sessions new, uncertain, and ambivalent. Such a member is dependent particularly on the leader and then on the other people for the warmth, acceptance, experiences, opportunities, guidance, and information which will help him use the group.

While each individual comes to the group with a 'transference' potential towards the other members the first relationship is with the leader. Because of the transference potential in the situation this tends to evoke the dependency of the earlier mother–child relationship. The mother is usually the first adult that the infant connects with and the quality of relationship established with 'mother' can be powerful in determining the quality of subsequent relationships. So from the start I accept the role of the 'mothering one' since I will usually be cast in a 'parenting' role anyway, and concern myself with the physical, emotional, and intellectual needs of the members in order to 'bond' with them. In this way I try to establish a firm and secure basis upon which each member can begin to move out into the group and engage with the other members.

I want to look at this now in relation to practice in the opening sessions of the group.

Nurturing at the physical level of group inclusion

Where possible I would suggest that you try to consider in advance how the environment will affect or constrain the group. Try to inspect and, if necessary, arrange the room you will work in so that it looks attractive and friendly. Consider: Is the room too big, too small? Will it permit people to move about during the course of their work? Is it warm and airy? How will people sound in this room? Can you be heard outside? Are you likely to be disturbed by external noises? Do you have to be careful with room furnishings or particular materials? Where are the toilets and kitchens?

Music, food, and names

As the group gathers for the first session I often play some suitable music in the background as I have found this a good way of 'warming' people and creates a friendly and welcoming atmosphere. I may also provide tea and biscuits as a traditional and sometimes practical method of nourishing people as well as giving them a means of gently easing into the group. Where possible try to seat the group comfortably in a circle as this allows each member to view the others and be seen. It also promotes optimum conversation and communication. Always greet people as they enter the room, go forward to welcome them, shake their hand and say their name if you know it, or ask them if you don't.

Exercise and games to break the ice

Think about using games or physical activity if appropriate as a way of relieving tension, getting people to contact each other, and facilitating interaction and communication. In the early sessions group members can be anxious, withdrawn, and wary of contact with each other. This can result in members blushing, inhibiting their breathing, and stiffening their posture in order to separate and defend themselves. The energy in the group can feel cold, staccato, and introverted. Well thought out physical activity can be useful, therefore, in releasing some of this inert energy and breaking the ice. It is important that any programme of activity at this stage is kept simple. A minimum of clear instructions will indicate what is expected of members and a minimal demand for skill competence will be more likely to engage members and promote success. There is a wide range of games and exercises specifically designed to 'accelerate' the process of inclusion and Chapter 10 contains a selection of activities and suggestions on how to use them.

Nurturing at the emotional level of group inclusion

Try to foster group cohesion and the development of trust from the start.

Group cohesion and the building of trust is a dynamic process which can be altered or changed by particular incidents, the strength of members' attraction to the group, and its relevance to their lives. Cohesion is a primary factor in keeping a group together and a major determinant of the quality of the climate and the effectiveness of the group. Cohesion develops through the acknowledgement of common elements so look for emotional themes and patterns in the early stages of the group. In this way you help people begin to see that they are not alone in feeling anxious or shy and they have more in common with other people than they at first realize. Concentrate on linking and connecting people by encouraging them to discuss and share whatever experiences they are having here and now in the group. Reward and reinforce any attempts by members to reach out towards each other. A way of doing this is to begin to develop desirable norms of behaviour.

Building group norms

Try to establish and promote those norms and values which will foster group cohesion. Here are some examples of relevant norms:

- Everybody is important and worthwhile in this group.
- As far as possible only one person at a time should speak.
- It is important that other members pay attention and listen.
- Do not judge people's behaviour. Try to discover the need behind or meaning of the behaviour.
- Group members will try to help each other sort out problems and difficulties.
- The sessions are to be kept confidential.

An easy way of developing positive norms in the beginning is to give the group permission to behave or feel in a certain way. A technique that I often use is to write certain permissions on sheets around the room such as:

- It's OK to make mistakes here.
- It's OK not to know here.
- I can ask for help here.

I then ask members to select one or two from the dozen or so cards, which they can use as their 'motto' for the session. You can also ask members to discuss why they chose a particular permission.

Another way of fostering desirable norms is to reinforce statements by members which will help the group accomplish its goals or maintain its emotional well-being such as, 'I think we should be honest about how we feel', or 'I think it would show commitment if we all agreed to come on time'.

Members will be more accepting of norms that they have set up so pay close attention to what people say they want and what they say will make them do certain things. When you know *what* will move people then you know *how* to move them.

Permit what is happening and acknowledge the real issues of concern

Allow whatever is happening to happen. Permit people to be silent or passive or shy. Do not force them into discussion or activity in order to fill up spaces or give the impression that this is a busy and therefore successful group. You may feel that you want to avoid embarrassing pauses and silences but by 'filling in' you may miss an opportunity to focus on what is really bothering people.

I have found that members are generally relieved and appreciative when I acknowledge how difficult it is to talk with people we hardly know. By drawing attention to those gaps in conversation in a warm and nurturing way you can make them normal and legitimate, and you can demonstrate to members that you understand and care about their ambivalence and tension about inclusion. It is then much easier than you would think to get people talking about their anxieties about speaking in public or fears about revealing too much of themselves.

In other situations members may talk too much; there may be a lot of repetitiveness or showing off. I will endeavour to point out how these behaviours may be a way of avoiding contact with other people, dealing with threatening silences, or forcing the leader to provide more structure. I take care to acknowledge the needs and fears as natural and only to be expected whenever people come together initially. I then try to help members explore why they feel like this in this particular group and look at what they can do about it.

Put events in context and make connections

Try to refer members to previous experiences of 'beginning' such as the first day in a new school or job, moving to a new neighbourhood, or making new friends. By '*contextualizing*' beginnings in this way you can help group members see their current inclusion experiences from a wider life perspective and this can desensitize the situation a great deal. Themes which often emerge at this stage include how people present themselves, poor self-image, fear of rejection, lack of confidence, fear of forming relationships with the opposite sex, and inadequacy in basic social skills. The purpose of the particular group will determine how much time you will spend discussing these themes. The important point to remember is that emotional needs and concerns about inclusion must be acknowledged and worked with if they are not to sabotage and undermine the group endeavour.

Do not force or insist on trust

Many group workers like to develop cohesion and trust in the group through the use of 'trust-games'. I do use these games but have sometimes seen them used in a way which can be injurious to the development of healthy group trust. Cohesion and trust develop in a group through members unfolding experiences and encounters with each other. This takes time and it is in the nature of things that trust should unfold, should be earned. Over-emphasis and insistence that group members *should* trust each other or *must* be more trusting can often indicate insecurity on the part of the worker, may come across as insincere and fraudulent, and can actually produce the opposite outcome. It is much better to establish cohesion and trust in the manner I have suggested – working directly out of members' behavioural and emotional expressions in a gentle, nurturing, and accepting way.

Establishing structure: the check-in

Gradually members come to see that there is a structure emerging in the group; that it is alright to have these feelings of anxiety or helplessness or ambivalence and that there exist ways of dealing with them. This gives a sense of definition and control which is reassuring and actually enhances conditions for increased risk-taking, disclosure, and the development of trust.

From the start of the group I try to develop a sense of structure and foster the emergence of consistency and predictability by assuming a firm and 'directive' stance which is compatible with and supplements my nurturing of the group. I will indicate when the sessions start, usually by asking people to 'check in'. This involves members individually connecting to the group by verbalizing how they are feeling, what they have done since last session, what they are anxious about, or looking forward to in this session. The check-in acknowledges the need to 'include' at the start of each session and builds in a structured nurturing and orienting period. It also gets each member to speak for a short time in a low stress situation since each individual can decide the length and content of their contribution.

Clearing expectations, contracting, routines

In the early sessions I will find out from each member what expectations they have of the group, what they want from the group, and why they have come. People tend to expect this and are usually happy to supply this information. Another method of establishing structure and control in these opening sessions is to negotiate a contract with members about what is and is not permissible (see page 99). Throughout the early sessions of the group I attempt to build a safe and stable context within which members can participate and interact successfully and with satisfaction. I am not afraid to arbitrate and make decisions, since members expect this of me. I do try to explain why I have chosen a particular course and look for comment and feedback on this, if appropriate.

Consistent patterns are important in building a sense of structure and orthodoxy and so I establish regular routines such as meal breaks, activities, check-ins, reviews, and planning periods which can be easily formalized and structured into group experience.

Do not be afraid to lead

I should emphasize that I am directing the group in a light and sensitive manner as a way of acknowledging and responding to people's need for structure and boundary. This directing is more in the sense of guiding or showing the way rather than imposing arbitrary rules on group members. I think it is very important that from the outset members can see that the leader is willing and confident in his ability to lead and guide the group. This instils confidence and trust in the leader and makes it easier to explore what the group has to offer.

Some group workers seem to expect members to 'take responsibility' for the structure of the group from the start, refusing to guide and direct on the grounds that 'it's your group'. In some instances this is to misunderstand the responsibility and nature of the authority vested in the group worker, seeing only the negative aspects of power and control; and worse, ignoring members' legitimate needs for direction from the group leader. The consequence can be to unwittingly turn the group into an unsafe and random experience where a form of jungle law predominates in the absence of a carefully designed boundary and structure.

Nurturing at the intellectual level of group inclusion

At the level of members' intellectual needs there are a number of issues to be aware of. Members will be curious about you and about each other, so creating space to satisfy this curiosity is essential. Because personal information and reasons for being in the group are often vague, superficial, or not fully absorbed in the tension and anxiety of having to speak publicly, I tend to use pairing-type exercises as a way of deepening and obtaining knowledge about each other. Making a short statement about myself from a more personal angle is a useful way of dispelling any reasonable curiosity about me and can always be augmented by allowing members to ask questions.

Clarifying purpose and making contracts

It is important that members focus on the purpose of the group, think about why they are here, and reflect on their commitment to the group goals. A way of doing this is to set aside time right from the start to clarify expectations. Do not be afraid to ask lots of questions in order to help people identify and make explicit their expectations, fantasies, and apprehensions about the group's purpose, its way of working, and their role in it:

- What do you think this group is for?
- Why have you come?
- What do you want for yourself from the group experience?
- What are you worried about?
- What do you need in order to be here?

This process can be enhanced by encouraging individuals to make personal contracts with you or the group. These personal contracts can range from how people intend to use the group, to telling you before they run out of the session. Make *lots* of these contracts. They are a very powerful way of clarifying people's desires and fears and eliciting and engaging their ability to determine for themselves.

Aim to arrive at a statement of what is realistic, possible, and desirable in this group which can be put to members in the form of a group contract. The group contract is vital to ensure that members understand what is being asked of them and can agree to pursue particular objectives. Articulation of goals at the individual and collective level develops consensus, motivates behaviour, and indicates tasks and performances as well as creating security and a sense of well-being.

It is important that the group contract is discussed fully and that members can interact and share ideas about the proposed goals and programme. Obviously this will vary from group to group. In one group there will be a clear and acceptable task and members will get down to work immediately. In another group, particularly those which emphasize more personal work, it may take several sessions to successfully negotiate why it is that people have come and what they expect and agree to do together.

Share your vision of the group

You can help a good deal by joining in and stating how you would like to see the group developing. Some workers see this stance as too directive or manipulative and prefer to withdraw to the sidelines to let the group decide its own purpose and direction. My own position is that since I am in the group for a particular reason and have an investment in it by virtue of my time, resource, and energy I have a professional right, if not an obligation on behalf of a funding agency, to seek a preferred and agreed purpose and direction. My experience is that people appear relieved, respond better, remain committed to the group task, and are more motivated when I am explicit and unambiguous about my wishes for the group and maintain no secret ambitions or hidden agendas.

In carefully putting out my vision of how the group might operate I aim to not only declare what I am unwilling or not prepared to undertake but also to stimulate discussion and begin to develop consensus as to what we are here for. If you decide to suggest possibilities and options for the group in order to help people identify their needs or make up their minds the important point to remember is that you must always allow individuals the space and respect to consider and decide for themselves how they will meet their needs.

You can promote respect, develop consensus, and facilitate the emergence of a healthy task and goal structure by ensuring that:

- Individuals understand your purpose in setting up the group/ working with the group.
- Can discuss this if necessary.
- Individuals can identify particular personal needs or problems that the group can help with.

- Individuals can see how other people can contribute to their circumstance and can see how they can reciprocate.
- There is minimum competition and maximum co-operation.
- Group goals are clear, feasible, and attractive.
- Group goals are relevant to individual needs.
- Individuals feel valued, significant, and listened to.
- You approach the business of goal-setting, group contracting, formulating programme, establishing rules and procedures with humour, common sense, and a willingness to negotiate with and involve people.

If you have been effective in working with the group at the levels of physical, emotional, and intellectual inclusion members will have been helped to make a decision to belong to the group and the group will feel as if it has an existence of its own. You will be able to tell if members have included themselves and whether or not the group is developing satisfactory levels of cohesion and trust because:

A high degree of cohesion is indicated by:	A low degree of cohesion is indicated by:
• Good attendance • Frequent meetings • Punctuality • Stable membership • Members like each other, are friendly, trusting, supportive, open • Members work well on tasks and goals • Group feels warm, humorous, and fun • Members adhere to group norms	• Absenteeism, poor or erratic attendance • Infrequent meetings, postponement, cancellations • Lateness, bad time-keeping • Turnover, loss or change of members • Members unfriendly, guarded, suspicious • Members compete with each other on tasks and goals • Group feels cold, strained, anxious • Members disregard group norms

Review

- Behaviour in the opening sessions of the group can be construed as the interplay of the love and will energies expressed individually and collectively in terms of basic needs for survival, safety, and membership. (Look at Maslow's hierarchy of needs on page 66 to see how his first three levels of need correspond to the inclusion stage.)

- Recurrent behaviour can indicate that individuals are assuming or are being assigned to roles which may be related more to personal need than to the task or goals of the group (see page 71).

- Recognition of the need motivating the behaviour or role is essential if intervention is to be appropriate.

- The group cannot evolve to its next stage of development until its basic needs have been met.

- This requires the leader to work with the group on the physical, emotional, and intellectual levels of its being.

- The leader assumes a nurturing and guiding stance in relation to group members.

- Irrespective of gender the leader assumes the role of the mothering one – the group mother.

- The leader fosters the development of trust and group cohesion.

- The leader seeks to establish structure and consistency within the group.

- The leader negotiates a contract with members which is explicit about the purpose of the group and the ways in which it will work.

Chapter 5

Work at the middle stages of the group: control issues

Just when members seem to have decided to invest in the group a change in atmosphere may occur which can at first be confusing and alarming to the more inexperienced group worker. Previously friendly or helpful individuals may suddenly reveal a less attractive side to their personality. Without warning the worker can find himself under attack, may be sabotaged, flouted, or even rejected; members start to fight with each other and everywhere there seems to be competition, conflict, and rebellion.

Despite the evidence to the contrary, what is happening in the group is in fact quite natural. The seeming chaos is simply another manifestation of the dynamic tension between the love and will energies which are always present in the group. The successful resolution of the inclusion stage has come about because the love principle has prevailed over the individuals' need to pull away from the group. Now the will principle begins to eclipse its twin as members get to grips with what it means to be in this group. The love principle begins to wane as members increasingly adjust to new roles and ways of functioning and start to explore and test collective, personal, and worker limitations and potentials. In other words the group is beginning to differentiate. Having made the decision to join in the group people are now trying to define and formalize relationships, mark out boundaries, and create a social structure.

This period is called the *control stage* because the problems of status, rank, competition, power, influence, and authority become dominant issues. The control stage represents a crucial period of transition from a less intimate to a more intimate system of relationships within the group and strange as it may seem the way in which intimacy is established is through competition and the struggle for leadership.

Underlying interaction at this stage are two central issues which each individual eventually has to confront:

- How much influence can I exercise in this group?
- How much personal autonomy do I have to give up to be in this group?

These two concerns generate the following types of questions in the minds of members:

- *The others*: Who are the influential and powerful members? Who is the most powerful? Where do I fit in? How much power have I got? Can I get more? What is the currency or medium for power and influence? Do I have to fight anyone here? How can I get on the winning side? Who should I support here?
- *The limits*: What are the rules in this group? Do I agree with them? Can I change them? Who makes the rules? What will happen if I break them? What sanctions and penalties are there? Who makes the decisions in this group? Will I be involved? How much will I be involved?
- *The leader*: Can I trust him? Is he dependable, reliable? Can he maintain control in the group? How will he handle conflict? Is he strong or weak? What will he do if I break the rules? Does he have favourites? Does he like me? Will he intervene in time?

During this stage of group life each group member experiences anxiety and tension about whether they have too much or not enough power and influence and whether they have too much or not enough personal freedom. In order to minimize this anxiety each group member behaves in a way which will create the degree of influence and autonomy that is most comfortable for him. This behaviour tends to be directed towards the leader and other group members, who can often experience these actions as skewed and distorted if not openly destructive.

The inexperienced group leader and members may react to attack or threat by fighting back or fleeing from the scene, succeeding often only in exacerbating the situation. The more experienced leader comprehends the 'fight or flight' nature of group behaviour and intervenes appropriately.

In some groups the actual period of disintegration may be slight and after spending some time exploring its functioning a group may make the necessary adjustments to its structure or goals and move on with its work. In other situations the struggle may be protracted or unresolved and the group can get stuck at this stage, regress to the previous stage, or in some extreme instances terminate. Before we go on to examine ways in which the worker can facilitate the group let us identify some of the more typical behaviours to be found at the control stage:

Moving away from or against other members (Will principle)	Underlying needs and motives
• Absences, lateness • Silence • Avoidance of issues/ members • Selfishness, refusal to share, compromise • Walking out of group • Drop-outs, ending of membership • Verbal or physical violence • Scapegoating, blaming others, excluding • Emergence of powerful or aggressive members • Monopolizing, dominating, character assassination • Development of sub-groups, cliques, alliances • Power struggles, jockeying for position, rivalry, competition, plots, conspiracies • Questioning, belittling the group	• Need to be valued, esteemed • Fear of being rejected • Need to exercise power, influence • Fear of being dominated, attacked, oppressed • Need to be separate, autonomous, independent • Need to protect self from more powerful members • Need to run away – engage in flight activity • Need to attack as a way of asserting, maintaining, or defending self • Need to join with other more or less powerful members • Need to determine rank, status position within the group

Moving away from or against the leader (Will principle)	Underlying needs, and motives
• Direct or indirect verbal attack	• Need to know leader can be trusted, relied on for protection, is competent
• Sabotage, undermining authority, rebellion, flouting rules	• Fear that leader will not be able to prevent group from disrupting completely
• Trying to provoke leader into anger, disapproval, rejection	• Is the leader strong or weak?
• Searching for evidence of inconsistent behaviour	• Is he clear about his values?
• Trying to get leader to side with an individual, sub-group	• Need to know what the leader's limits are
• Looking for evidence of favouritism, special treatment	• How much rebellion will he permit?
• Testing leader's commitment to group goals, contracts, rules	• How much control will he allow members over their own affairs?
	• Need to assert self and be independent of the leader
	• Need to 'kill the father'
	• Existence of positive or negative transference

Fathering: leading the group at the control stage

If the worker is to sensitively guide the group through the control stage it is essential that he adopt a stance which facilitates the needs and objectives manifesting in individual and collective behaviour at this time. Although the confusion and inconsistency of this stage can appear most bewildering to the beginning group worker it is in fact within certain bounds essential for group development as a way of establishing for group members:

- A sense of self-control and adequacy.
- An ability to initiate one's own activity.

- Competence in the physical, social, and intellectual requirements of the group.
- Power, status, and the leadership in the group.

Moving towards other group members (Love principle)	Underlying needs and motives
• Pairing behaviours	• To interact, be part of, connect
• Expression of sexual attraction	• To be valued, affirmed, esteemed
• Sub-group formation	
• Compromising, sharing, agreeing, rules and norms	• To be protected, feel secure, have order, system, consistency, and predictability
• Consensual decision-making	
• Resolution of conflicts	• To influence, exercise power in a positive way
• Joining in activity	

The worker's ability to tolerate and permit a degree of rebellion is absolutely crucial if members are to successfully negotiate this stage. Unfortunately many workers do not fully understand what is happening in the group at this time and fiercely resist any attempts by members to diverge from the worker's wishes.

It is worth saying a little about this. In my experience of supervising workers, the control stage of group development causes most confusion, worry, and fear for the beginner and even for the not-so-new leader. The physical and emotional noise, violence, and hostility which can be met with at this stage is often quite frightening to the novice and almost always is construed as a reflection on his personal and professional competence.

Just why it is that a worker comes to see a group's behaviour as a threat to his image of himself as a worker is very interesting. One major factor is that most new workers would appear to have a fantasy of how a group should behave and how the ideal leader should operate. This fantasy has been built up from readings about the successful and glamorous interventions of accomplished group workers. Perhaps the worker has seen films of groups run in a children's home or an American drug addiction centre or has even had some positive experience himself in a professionally run group. When the worker's own ego needs to be helpful, esteemed, and successful are added to this pastiche, the result can be to create quite definite impressions, assumptions, and expectations of how a group and its leader should behave. Very rarely is the worker able to acknowledge the unreality of the role he has mentally reserved for himself or for members.

Faced with the sometimes ugly and painful reality of the group they are working with, most leaders amazingly prefer to preserve their idealized image and conclude that either something is wrong with the group or that they are obviously inadequate as a leader! Both conclusions are usually gross distortion and most unhelpful to a group which is struggling with very real and substantive issues of power and autonomy.

Frequently I see a beginning worker make one of two decisions. Some workers decide that it is their *personal responsibility* to make the group succeed in spite of deviant members. Since their way of doing this is to make the group conform to rules and the leader's personal authority the result is to initiate a spiral of ever-increasing repression, counter-sabotage, and inhibition. Other workers decide that they are inadequate in the circumstances and not cut out to be a group worker. They may slide into a paralysis which frightens group members who behave even worse in a vain attempt to engage the leader in some effort to direct and control. When this is not forthcoming the group can degenerate into panic, chaos, and ultimately termination.

What these workers are failing to see is that the struggles between members or sub-groups or with the leader is an expression of the way in which each member resolves the anxiety and tension generated in establishing the degree of influence and autonomy that is most comfortable for him. Inevitably the style of leading adopted by the worker is out of gear with the needs of members and only adds to the group's problems. What is actually needed is a philosophy and style of working with the group which provide clear direction and control and yet permit a degree of rebellion in which individual autonomy and influence can develop.

I believe this can be done only when the worker 'recognizes and accepts the members' need to see him as the group father'.

Earlier I likened the inclusion stage of group process to the stage of infancy and childhood watched over by the nurturing mother, and developing the analogy, the control stage corresponds more to that period of adolescence which is characterized by the association and supremacy of the peer group and rebellion against the authority of the 'father', however actual or symbolic.

The world of the adolescent is increasingly the world of the 'father' – the external world of role and responsibility, power and influence, status and prestige. The adolescent is at once attracted to this world because of what it offers and repelled because it threatens to curtail and inhibit him through the operation of the greater power of the father. And yet each individual finds himself moving away from dependence on the mother and a more introverted world and seeking an image of himself as a unique, autonomous, and influential person. Vital to this process is the way in which the individual manages the significant social relationships of the peer group and the model of authority and leadership presented to him initially through his struggles with the father.

What group members need from their leader at this stage is not repressive conformity to rules or the other extreme of paralysis but the understanding, permission, firmness, and protection that come from acknowledging their need to challenge and seek for power and discover their impact on authority. Put another way what members need from a leader at this stage is for him knowingly to take on their projections and become the 'group father'.

By taking on the role of group father the worker clearly signals to the members his willingness to be in an authority relationship with members – but one which has individual and collective interests at heart. The leader indicates that he will permit members to challenge him for a share in leadership but that he will not allow them to disrupt the group completely. He will not take total responsibility for the operation of the group because that would only foster an unnatural dependency; but he can be relied on and trusted in the struggle for self-sufficiency. As group father the leader will be available to support, encourage, and help each member, and he will agree to exercise restraint in the use of his power in order to help each member connect to their own authority.

There are a number of tasks that the group father must accomplish at this stage.

Role of the group father at the emotional level

Permit what is happening to occur

We have seen this before (see page 96). Do not assume that you always have to intervene in an argument or fight between members or that you must always respond to provocative behaviour. It is vital that you are on guard against taking responsibility which belongs to the group, particularly when the limits and boundaries are being tested. Often members will attempt to induce you to act in an authoritarian way which will allow them to slide along relatively uninvolved or force you to structure or set the limits.

Acknowledge that you can see something happening. Let them know you have got the message but do not necessarily jump in. Let the situation develop a little if you can, in order to see what is really going on or to think about an appropriate response. By allowing what is happening, you encourage members to express themselves more freely and indicate that you expect them to begin assuming more responsibility for themselves and negotiate their own solutions.

Provide protection and support where necessary

Clearly there are times when what is occurring in the group is actually or potentially hazardous or injurious. In these instances you may decide that it is appropriate for you to intervene in order to assure the physical or emotional safety of an individual or the group. While you might attract ridicule or hostility for your intervention usually the group is secretly quite relieved and reassured that you are prepared to come to someone's aid.

When members know that you can be relied on in these times of crisis or emergency they are encouraged to be more open and take greater risks in relationship. This has major implications for the development of a more respectful and egalitarian structure in the group since the presence of appropriate protective controls tends to inhibit jungle law and the emergence of hierarchies.

A situation which often appears to demand the use of protective controls is the presence of a scapegoat in the group. Before rushing in to protect the scapegoat it is important to evaluate the situation thoroughly if you are not to actually make it worse.

Scapegoating usually involves the displacement or transfer of anger from its real object onto a weaker and more acceptable target. Much scapegoating occurs in groups where members do not feel able or safe to attack the leader and so they vent their anger on a weaker member. Certain members seem to be more likely to be scapegoated than others:

- Anyone who emphasizes their difference from other people whether it be sickness, weakness, or superiority.
- Anyone who openly expresses what the group is trying to avoid.
- Anyone who provokes in a manner inviting attack or victimization.

While these people attract hostility in their own right they are often attacked only because members are reluctant to direct their anger to where it really belongs. So when preparing to protect or support a scapegoat check to see if you are in actuality the real target of aggression or whether anger should be redirected towards a very dominant or able group member. If this is the case it might be more appropriate to describe what you think is really happening. In this way you can help the group express itself more realistically and then begin to help the involved parties understand the curious and ambiguous relationship between victim and persecutor.

In other situations you can protect and support in subtle ways. Shy people or members who find it hard to speak up can be more easily encouraged if you sit facing them where you can give them non-verbal cues without interrupting the conversation. You can support those people who want to be thought of as leaders in the group by sitting close to them. Applaud and compliment people when they deserve it and try to praise the act rather than the person as this comes over much more sincerely and avoids embarrassment and confusion.

Members can very easily get depressed and discouraged at this stage and will often ask if they are the worst group you have ever worked with or whether you consider them bad or even mad! While they may or may not be the all-time low, it is important that you reassure them that their struggles and conflicts, questions and doubts are really quite natural at this period in a group's life. Only then can you begin to refocus their attention and get them to look at the underlying power issues which so strongly motivate their behaviour.

Role of the group father at the intellectual level

Clarify the issues when you intervene

In deciding whether to intervene in a particular situation try as far as possible to understand the needs and motives of the people concerned and the position of the group so that you can focus on what is really happening (see page 95). Much behaviour is an individual or collaborative manoeuvre to engage the leader, avoid involvement, or appear significant and it will be important to address the deeper meanings of these actions if members are to begin to express themselves more appropriately and articulately.

Whether you know what is happening or not you may sometimes feel that you just have to act immediately to prevent or proscribe behaviour but usually most situations will, on reflection, allow you several other choices.

- You can allow the situation to continue in the expectation that other members will eventually become so impatient, bored, or restless that they will deal with it. You can then intervene or not to examine what was taking place and promote insight and learning.
- You can ask the group why they are letting this situation develop.
- You can ask the people involved what it is that they really need in the group at this time.
- You can ask the people involved and the group to help you look at what is happening.

Any one of these choices will help to focus the group on the *process* of their interaction and begin to identify and articulate the real issues of concern for the group.

Although Chapter 9 contains suggestions on how you might teach a group to analyse its own process at any period of its life I think it would be valuable to look at a simple sequence which will help you clarify the various issues at the control stage. Obviously it will help if you have carefully cultivated throughout an attitude that difficulties and differences are natural and that group members should be concerned for each other and willing to stay with problems and work them out.

- A situation may recur or be identified which you believe needs to be properly explored. Try to identify a specific behaviour or pattern that you can focus on: a particular conflict; repeated avoidance and distraction by members when asked to concentrate on a topic; flouting of a certain rule, or belittling the purpose of the group.
- Identify who is involved and when:

> One individual versus another
> An individual versus you, the leader
> An individual versus a sub-group/whole group
> Sub-group/group versus you

- Identify the needs and the values *you* wish to preserve at this time. Here are some of them:

> Your need to provide good leadership
> Your need to maintain the group's well-being
> Your need to help the group be productive
> Your need to protect standards

- Try to identify the needs and values of the participants. They will centre around:

> Members' need to be affirmed as worthwhile
> Members' need to be accepted and included
> Members' need for influence
> Members' need for autonomy

- Try to find some needs or values that you and the people concerned have in common.
- Decide if it is appropriate for you to intervene.
- Make a short statement about what you see happening. You might want to say how you feel about this, or what effect you see this behaviour having on the group. Talk about the values

you have in common and say *why* you want to look at what is happening. Try to give people reasons to say *yes* to you – reasons that are to their or the group's advantage.

- Ask if people are prepared to look at the issues involved. When doing this try to ask questions which will engage people and elicit a 'yes' answer: 'You do want the group to work, don't you?' 'You want to get on with the activity, don't you?' 'You want to enjoy the group, don't you?' If people are unwilling to look at the issues don't push it at this stage because you might only exacerbate the situation or build opposition. Leave this responsibility with the group, knowing that they may change their mind or more likely the situation will recur again. Situations which are unfinished nearly always recur in the group and the next time you can legitimately put out some ultimatums.

  If you decide to issue an ultimatum, place it firmly in the context of the group contract that everyone agreed to. I find this a very effective way of depersonalizing the situation and invoking powerful reasons why this episode should be concluded. People find it very difficult to keep avoiding when you balance the issue against the purpose of the group or a contract that they freely entered into.

- Assuming you have agreement to explore the issue, invite contributions towards a mutual definition of the problem. Avoid tendencies to make the issue personal, blame others, or seek revenge. Try to get people to make statements about what they really *need* in the situation and watch for openings that permit you to respond to people's needs.

- Help the group consider the consequences of the behaviour in terms of costs and gains. This is important if you are to encourage members to identify the desirable or undesirable outcomes and make agreements or decisions about what to do.

  Do not be discouraged if you find that events occur too quickly or explosively in your group for you to use this model as you might like. Members may resist or you may find it nearly impossible to identify your own needs in the situation let alone theirs! With practice, and most importantly, by continually expecting group members to work on their problems you will find that you and the group are increasingly able to disengage from the struggle and begin to work more creatively on areas of common concern.

Encourage effective problem solving

Many groups founder at the control stage because they are unable or unwilling to resolve their problems.

Some of the reasons for this are:

- Lack of clarity in understanding the problem
- Lack of clarity in presenting the problem
- Not enough information
- A critical, overly evaluative, or competitive climate
- Interpersonal conflict or tension
- Pressures to conform
- Lack of motivation or interest
- Haste, urgency, or fear
- Ineffective or immature problem-solving skills
- Lack of leadership

Part of the role of the worker as group father is to inculcate in the group those norms and values which support the collaborative resolution of problems and difficulties. You must be explicit in your expectations that members will agree to seek solutions to their problems and will concur that a threat or difficulty for even one member immediately becomes a *community affair* involving the collective well-being. Only if these attitudes are present will the group be motivated enough to focus on their affairs.

Often I find that a group needs assistance or training in order to use inquiry and problem-solving methods to advantage. In these situations I use a simple five-stage model to teach the group the necessary processes:

1   Identifying the problem
2   Analysing the problem
3   Drawing up alternative strategies
4   Selecting a strategy
5   Evaluation

These stages can be very effectively taught by doing a 'force-field' analysis on a particular problem. Basically what this means is that most problem situations can be understood in terms of forces that push towards improvement and forces which hinder this movement. By identifying the 'helping' forces and the 'restraining' forces it is possible to generate a number of points which will permit intervention in order to produce change.

The most difficult part of the whole problem-solving process for the group is making a clear, reliable, and accurate statement of the problem. The discussion in the previous section on how to clarify the issues in a particular situation will help you negotiate an agreed definition of the problem and elicit a commitment to work on it.

The next step is to conduct the force-field analysis in order to determine the nature and magnitude of the various forces involved in the problem. To do this, involve the group in making lists of all the restraining forces and then all the helping forces. Try to do this without prejudice or criticism.

Review each list and rank the forces according to their importance in affecting the problem. Identify the more important restraining forces and list some possible methods of reducing or eliminating each one. Turn to the helping forces and make a list of ways in which the effect of each helping force could be increased.

The third step in problem solving is to draw up alternative strategies. Force-field analysis is a particularly useful way of drawing up alternative strategies for solving a problem because it gives three options:

1	Increase strength or number of helping forces
2	Decrease strength or number of restraining forces
3	Simultaneously increase helping forces while decreasing restraining forces

It is important to review the group problem in the light of each of these options and discuss which is most promising. Look for the positive and negative consequences of each option and add any new steps that will expand the alternative and make it more successful. Ensure that everyone participates and is listened to and that those who disagree are allowed to express themselves.

Once all the possible options have been drawn up and discussed, the group needs to select the strategy it will implement. This procedure involves the group in decision making which is fully explored in the next section. In selecting an appropriate strategy the following points might be helpful:

* Select the most promising alternatives and weigh up the positive advantages in adopting each one
* Cost each strategy in terms of time, resource, money, people, etc.
* Weigh up the likely benefits against the cost of implementation
* Try to anticipate possible obstacles and impediments
* Choose the most viable strategy
* Identify and assign roles and responsibilities for implementing strategy
* Initiate the strategy

The final step in problem solving is to evaluate the success of the strategy in terms of bringing about the desired outcome. Sometimes solving one problem often brings other problems into the open and the whole sequence has to be repeated for a new situation. Again the desired outcome may not be achieved and the group will have to develop and try new strategies until they find one that is effective. In evaluating these circumstances it is important to reinforce the idea of problem solving as a process which is continually evolving and unfolding rather than as a static, fixed point affair, if you are to help the group guard against depression, futility, and inadequacy.

I like to foster effective problem solving and provide the group with plenty of practice by combining exercises and simulations designed to develop problem-solving skills, with appropriate difficulties thrown up by their real-life interaction and attempts at achieving the group task. In this way members learn procedures and acquire confidence and dexterity in handling uncertainty, settling their own affairs, and dealing with problematic situations. If you wish to use an exercise or simulation to promote problem-solving skills with your group you can find some examples and suggestions in Chapter 10.

Here are ways to encourage effective problem solving.

- Make the problem specific, clear, and simple
- Make it to people's advantage to solve the problem
- Expect members to be involved
- Discourage defensiveness, blaming, criticism
- Make the problem a communal one
- Ensure everyone gets a fair hearing
- Discourage coalitions or alliances which block or stifle other members
- Focus on those aspects of the problem which can be solved
- Make space for members to express their feelings
- Bring conflicts and disagreements out into the open
- Encourage creative and divergent thinking
- Combine ideas where possible
- Summarize the group's progress at intervals
- Ensure everyone feels ready to make choices, decisions
- Ensure everyone feels committed to decision or solution

Promote decision making

Like problem solving the process of decision making is a fundamental feature of group life. In order to achieve anything every group needs a method of determining and setting about its objectives. This is the function of decision making which in its simplest sense means initiating proposals and securing agreement to do something.

It almost always involves a choice between several different possibilities and this immediately creates a power dimension because frequently there can develop a spread of competing desire and interest amongst members. When we remember that each member at the control stage of group development is concerned with his position and influence it becomes apparent how bound up decision making is with the core issues of power, influence, and authority.

Decision making can come to be viewed by members as a way of engaging in the ongoing power struggles, acting aggressively, gaining in personal significance and esteem. The way in which the group resolves its control issues through the decision-making process in this phase will determine whether or not the group will be able to survive and work in any meaningful fashion and so facilitating and teaching effective decision making is a primary concern of the worker at this time.

There are a number of ways in which a group can reach a decision and each is appropriate in certain situations:

- Agreement (consensus) of the whole group
- Majority vote
- Decision of the member with most expertise
- Decision of the member with most authority

Of these, I believe the most effective method of group decision is by consensus. It also takes the most time. Consensus means that everyone agrees what the decision should be and feels that they have been involved. Consensus is reached when each member understands and is prepared to support the decision. Even those members who may have had differing views will be prepared to give the decision support for an experimental period of time.

To achieve consensus takes time because all members must be encouraged to state their views and, in particular, their opposition to other people's views. This can be a lengthy and at times conflictive process but is essential if each member is to feel he has been listened to with respect and has had a fair opportunity to influence the outcome. Here are some guidelines for developing consensual decision making in your group.

- Try to involve everyone in the discussion and decision making.
- Look for and bring into the open disagreements and differences of opinion. They are natural and to be expected. If properly used they are very helpful in widening the range of information and opinions, developing creativity and inventiveness.

  Do not avoid conflict and settle for easy options like majority vote or tossing a coin! Encourage people to see conflict as *part* of what goes on in groups and as healthy when dealt with in the open.
- Insist that people listen carefully to each other, accord each other basic respect and courtesy, particularly where they disagree or clash. Avoid blaming, scapegoating, unpleasant personalizing of discussion.

- Discourage rigid and fundamental position taking. Encourage members to explore underlying assumptions and to examine issues and facts.

- Because decisions are best based on facts, ideas, and values ensure that the relevant information is available and people know what values are at stake. In this way members can become aware of the reasons for their choices.

- Do not accept a stalemate position. Look for the next most acceptable alternative which will engage all members. This might mean working through various preferences until the dissenting or disputing factions can find one that offers the possibility of resolving the position with honour and without losing face. At times this may involve an element of *compromise* where each side may give a little in order to progress.

   At other times it is possible to create or invent a new possibility into which both sides can fit and be respected. When this happens the resulting integration can be very exciting and may open up new horizons for the group.

- At all times provide support for any member who wishes to make a contribution.

Decision making is a very dynamic process and one which will involve you closely with group members in sorting out possible alternatives and anticipating consequences. Try, where possible, to avoid making decisions for the group but rather give members as much practice and experience as they can tolerate in handling their own affairs. Members need to know that they have a right to make decisions and that you accept and safeguard their right to autonomy. As you encourage this, decision making will become more rational, less impulsive and egocentric, and more group-oriented.

If you wish to structure part of the group programme to provide opportunities to practise decision-making skills turn to Chapter 10 for some simple exercises and suggestions.

Role of the group father at the physical level

Using programme therapeutically

One prime way you can influence norms and encourage the behaviours you desire at this stage of group development is through the planning of programme activities (see page 31 and Chapter 10).

With some individuals or groups, for example, you may need to provide opportunities to release aggression in a controlled way.

Individuals may need to attain a sense of mastery or control over their own bodies or the environment. Activities such as chess, dance, art, or craftwork can satisfy this need and prevent its manifesting in the form of bullying or vandalism. Members' needs to compete, test authority, or overwhelm can be carefully channelled with a little thought or simply by asking the group what they could do.

I have indicated in the previous section how you can promote problem-solving and decision-making skills by using simulations and exercises, and you can, for example, cultivate sharing or co-operation by increased use of teamwork or activities which directly reward shaping behaviours. In another situation you may decide that the conflict or chaos in the group is a result of poor or inadequate communication skills. You can then devise a sequence of activity which will aim to build up the required repertoire. This need not be as complicated as you may think. A game like mimes or charades can be very effective in developing attending and concentration skills and non-verbal ability in a fun way.

The worker's role in this phase is to help group members to begin to relate to each other in an increasingly sophisticated and considerate manner. Since members need assistance to do this in most groups you need to give time to planning how you will use the programme to deal with the particular problems or conflicts that crop up. But do not feel that this is *your* responsibility exclusively. It is also important to help members perceive that group experience is something which they can modify in some degree to achieve particular ends and outcomes.

Review

- Control stage of group process is like the period of adolescence.
- Behaviour at this stage reflects each member's attempt to establish an optimum degree of influence and autonomy.
- Members need clear direction and control and yet must be allowed an appropriate degree of rebellion.
- The worker needs to adopt a style of leading which facilitates these issues.
- The metaphor of the group father is a way of engaging and activating the qualities and attributes of the will principle.

- The worker engages in a series of tasks with the group designed to identify, acknowledge, and resolve the power control issues of members.

Chapter 6

Work at the later stages of the group: affection issues

Following some resolution of the various control issues the group is now usually ready to settle down to work on its tasks and goals, whether this be dealing with the personal problems and anxieties of members in the therapeutic setting or defining a job and making plans to achieve it in the work group.

This impulse towards a more mature use of the group energy and resource comes about because of the emergence of an interpersonal structure which is supportive of group activity and concerned to further the best interests of members. What has happened is that individuals have come together to form a group; they have organized themselves in terms of responsibility and power and now they are ready to explore what it means to be emotionally involved with each other.

We can view the transition from the turbulence of the control stage to the relatively more cohesive and mature experience of this latest phase of group life as yet another manifestation of the dynamic tension between the ever-present love and will energies in the group. Under the aegis of the will principle the important structural issues of power, leadership, status, and position have been confronted and resolved to an appropriate degree. Now the love principle comes to predominate and relationships and alignments between members become based more on personal affection, mutual interest, or other attractions and less on consideration of strength, power, and influence.

There is a developing sense of 'we' or 'us' and members are more concerned to seek agreement or approval from each other than from the worker as previously. You can see this quite clearly in those instances where one member brings along a friend to a session and suggests he is eligible to join the group. The antagonisms and jealousies expressed towards the new person and his sponsor in such statements as, 'He won't know how we do things in this group', 'I can trust everybody here but I don't know him', 'Why do you want him here?' 'What's wrong with us?' and the threats to leave the group or be less active if the new person gets in all show the emergence of a new degree of in-group feeling, cohesion, and personal involvement. In other instances the appearance of imitative or idiosyncratic behaviour in dress, language, seating arrangements, and so on reveals more explicit agreement, identification, and group harmony.

As the group assumes more importance for members they work together often and more effectively and in turn this clarifies and stabilizes relationship patterns. With the passage of time there is more open acknowledgement of personal needs and prerogatives, mutual acceptance, and support. Because the group environment is becoming more permissive and caring there is more tolerance of individual differences and a heightened sense of personal identity; members increasingly come to differentiate between each other as unique persons. This can prove to be both an exciting and painful experience because members may be more explicit about their positive and negative feelings for each other and this can generate jealousy and hostility. However, the process of clarifying and coming to terms with intimacy gradually creates the freedom and ability to be different and acceptable if not always likeable.

As roles become more flexible and group energy is increasingly channelled into task activities you may observe among members, a growing ability to plan and carry out projects relevant to the purpose of the group. While there is a high degree of integration, consensus over tasks, and a thrust towards goal satisfaction, there may occur episodic conflicts and dissatisfactions as a result of particular crises faced by individuals. Generally, however, members are more aware of the relationship between group experience and personal growth and are usually well able to work through any crisis.

It is important that you look for interaction which revolves around these three clear issues:

- Being liked and being close
- The quality and satisfaction of work
- Individuality

These issues will generate questions and concerns for members such as the following.

Being liked and being close

Do the others like me? How much do they like me? Are the people I like interested in me? Do I have rivals for one person's affections? How close do I want to be to specific others in the group? How close will they permit me to come?

The quality and satisfaction of work

Do we work well together? Am I satisfied with the way we work and the results we achieve? Can the work be improved? What are the best means of achieving my/our goals? Is the work exciting, stimulating, demanding enough for me?

Individuality

Can I be different from the others and still be liked/accepted? Can I be more myself and still be liked/accepted? Will the group constrain me in any way? What opportunities does the group offer me to explore and discover new experiences, resources, abilities, and skills?

These underlying concerns will manifest in certain typical behaviours at this stage. (See pages 126–7.)

Guiding the group at the affection stage

If the inclusion stage of the group is analogous to infancy and the control stage to adolescence, then the affection stage can be said to resemble early adulthood and subsequent maturity in that members are less self-absorbed and more other-centred.

They are willing to give more of themselves, get on with each other, and work co-operatively on the goals of the group. Quite clearly an ethical system, social etiquette, and culture unique to the group can be seen to be emerging which suggests a developing maturity and self-confidence. This has obvious implications for the worker's relationship with members and the scale of his activity in the group.

Moving towards other group members (Love principle)	Underlying needs and motives
• Imitative behaviour, dress, language • Appearance of we/us/ our words • Less leader-centred, more group-centred • Emergence of more stable relationships – pairings, triads and sub-groups • Cohesiveness and identity • Humour, joking, teasing • Sharing of opinions • More immediate expression of personal feelings • Confrontation, jealousy • Increasing self-revelation • Increasing self-awareness • Dismantling of facades and images • More tolerant, caring atmosphere • Emergence of other-centred values and ethics: compassion, altruism, idealism, love, service, desire to care/ support, religious sentiment, etc. • Emergence of a world view, growing awareness of social, political, and international issues as they affect group life	• To connect and belong • To be liked and sought out by other members • To be regarded as significant, valuable, worthwhile • To give affection to others • To be of service to others • To be authentic and genuine • To share, support

Moving with or for other group members (Will principle)	Underlying needs and motives
• Increased generativity, ideas, suggestions, proposals • Increased productivity – projects, tasks • Interdependence, team-work, sharing, co-operative ventures • Emergence of task-centred roles, a division of labour • Flexibility and creativity • Individualism in behaviour, values • Ability to differentiate between members, acceptance of the individual	• To be generative • To be productive • To contribute • To be regarded as significant and valuable • To co-operate • To individuate

You may recall that at the inclusion stage, members needed help to deal with issues of attachment and *dependency*, and the 'mothering' or nurturing stance of the worker was designed to facilitate this. As the group moved into its control stage the major issues for members centred around power and *independence* and the worker responded by adopting the role of 'group father' which permitted a degree of rebellion while maintaining boundary and purpose.

Now the members are beginning to explore the opportunities and potential for involvement and *interdependence* and require from the worker an approach which permits and enhances group functioning on its own behalf. In practice, this means the worker begins to move into a less central role and encourages the group to do more of its own work. This does not mean that the worker abandons the group to its own devices or retires, comfortable in the expectation that members should now be entirely self-sufficient. The group members still need the worker although in a much more subtle and sophisticated way than previously.

At this stage of its life the group is increasingly in tune with its purpose and senses clearly the steps to be taken which will fulfil this purpose. Difficulties and crises still arise of course and the group requires from the worker a style and quality of intervention which will direct its awareness and mobilize its energy towards resolution of its problems.

An image which I find useful to employ in sustaining my intervention and activity at this stage is that of the 'guide'. A distinct impression of 'journey' can often spontaneously emerge in the group at this time and may be revealed in behaviour and language such as 'we've come a long way together', 'who would have thought we could get this far', 'we've come this far together, we might as well stick it out'. The idea of the guide as someone who journeys with, and facilitates the process of journeying can be very appealing and helpful.

Assuming the perspective and stance of the guide enables me to create a context in which I can consistently be available to members without interfering or over-involving myself in the very necessary process of the group finding its way. It evokes for me ideas of gentleness and compassion and suggests a style of intervening which aims to stimulate and develop a sense of knowing, of inner authority, or rightness at the personal and collective levels. And in times of crisis the stance of guide reminds me to actively encourage members to open up to a deeper awareness of self and find resolution and meaning by sharing and using individual and group resource.

The central aspect of the guide stance is perhaps the idea of 'service' implicit in the worker's actions at this stage of group life. For me the image of the guide speaks very directly to a quality of 'presence' manifested by the worker with the intention of unselfishly helping the group achieve increasing integration and become more functional. It provides a practical and conceptual framework which permits me to engage and influence the potential of the group for intimate, productive, and compassionate activity in the best interests of everyone.

We have seen that members are less self-absorbed and more other-centred, more generative and productive at this time and it is also my experience that group members actively seek out experiences which bring with them an awareness of human inter-dependence and the value of loving and serving one's fellow-man. Members will look for opportunities and ways of making compassionate responses to each other and clearly demonstrate a need to support and be of service. It is in this area that the 'service' aspect of the guide's role is most important.

Where possible I endeavour to mobilize and channel the group energy and potential for caring and connecting, and model for members a way of being which seeks to serve the best interests of all. In practice, this means that I look for those incidents or episodes which permit me to advance the value of sharing or working together to build a context in which meaning or resolution can emerge, and which demonstrates the lack of creativity and goodwill involved in manipulating or over-whelming each other.

Typically, I engage in behaviour which appears to be:

- Encouraging, stimulating, inspiring.
- Nurturing, supportive, allowing.

Often these behaviours are less discreet than they appear here and the more common occurrence is a continuum of worker activity that can be said to be distinctly guiding in style and effect. The guide then is a worker who is not caught up in the struggles and striving of the group but one who unselfishly offers a practical vision of how the group can interact and allows members to internalize it at their own pace, build on, and develop it in their own fashion.

I want now to explore in more detail how the worker manifests this 'practical vision' at the affection stage.

Guiding at the physical level of group affection

Intimacy and high group cohesion at this stage can develop out of members working together in a manner which is both satisfying and productive. It is important therefore that you pay attention to group activity and procedures at the physical or structural level in order to ensure that there is a unity between people's desires and how they go about achieving them. Look carefully at your group and ask yourself:

1	Are there clear goals?	p. 18
2	Are members committed to these clear goals?	p. 99
3	Do these clear goals allow for co-operation?	p. 100
4	Is there an appropriate level of trust, cohesion, and support?	p. 101
5	Are there effective decision-making procedures?	p. 118
6	Are there effective problem-solving procedures?	p. 115
7	Is there distributed participation and leadership?	p. 134
8	Is there constructive management of power and conflict?	p. 106
9	Is there effective communication of ideas and feelings?	p. 131
10	Is there a culture which fosters collaboration and teamwork?	p. 130

If you were able to answer yes to each question posed in the box above then you have a successful group and a very effective team of people. If you were unable to answer yes to each question then you need to think about ways of promoting teamwork and the next section will be of interest to you. You might also need to review earlier chapters which cover these various features.

Promoting teamwork

Promoting teamwork in this context means that the group must learn to see itself as a team rather than as a set of individuals. In a team people are aware of each other's strengths and weaknesses and will seek to act in a way which uses their diversity to serve the collective as well as the individual. In a team set-up, problems which arise are seen as confronting the group as a whole and not just separate individuals. Team thinking results in the group seeing itself as a pool of communal resource to be deployed whenever new forms of involvement are required or situational needs demand.

To assess the quality of teamwork at this stage I ask myself two basic questions:

- Does the group have the necessary skills and structures to work together co-operatively and effectively?

- Does the group have the relevant attitudes, values, and norms which encourage and support the use of these skills and structures?

The answers I obtain based on my observations and experience of the group help me to decide how much time and energy I need to invest in teaching collaborative skills or developing a teamwork ethic or both.

Let us look now at some of the skills and values needed to work as a team that we have not encountered before.

Fostering communication

Effective communication is a fundamental prerequisite for every aspect of group functioning. In particular, the co-operative activity so characteristic of this stage demands that people are able and willing to exchange information competently, co-ordinate their actions, and reach some understanding of each other. Usually communication is adequate because the worker has endeavoured to create good communication habits and procedures from the start of the group, but it can frequently happen that methods of communication which were acceptable at earlier stages of development need reworking now. This is because the emergence of more sophisticated collaborative activity requires a corresponding evolution in group and personal communication techniques.

If this is apparent my habit is to wait for an incident or crisis which reveals or results in a fracture of communication. I then frame the problem as one which has implications for us all and as a communal affair therefore requires members to teamwork to find the factors which contributed to or were involved in the breakdown. Usually the group is able to identify one or more of the following.

Factors interfering with communication process

- Prejudices ⎫
- Attitudes ⎬ on part of receiver or sender
- Clarity of message
- Appropriateness of message
- Ability to understand message
- Ability to respond to message
- Defensive behaviour
- Environmental distractions

Having identified the relevant factors the next step in the process is to develop a short programme using exercises and experiential activities to correct any skill deficiencies. Depending on the need this programme can run over part of the session, one or two sessions, or even longer.

I tend to focus on three distinct skills of communication at this stage:

1 Sending messages effectively.
2 Receiving messages effectively.
3 Giving feedback.

In Chapter 10 there are examples of exercises which will help develop these skills but for now I want to present the basic teaching points that need to be conveyed to members.

Sending messages effectively

- Take responsibility for messages by clearly owning them
- Make messages clear, simple, and specific
- Make verbal and non-verbal messages agree with each other
- Look for feedback about the meanings being attached to your message
- Repeat messages until understood
- Make the message and its medium appropriate
- Try to avoid judging or interpreting

Receiving messages effectively

- Indicate your desire to understand the message
- Avoid judging, interrupting, imposing solutions, or finishing the message for sender
- Restate the message in your own words and to the sender's satisfaction
- Check your perception of sender's message
- Negotiate an agreement about the real meaning of the message if necessary

Giving feedback

- Give feedback as soon as you can after a particular behaviour or incident
- Make your feedback concrete and specific
- Describe your own feelings about the event but avoid judging or moralizing
- Look for and allow other perceptions and reactions
- Do not give a superficial answer or statement. If you have nothing to say – say so

While teaching members these skills will undoubtedly facilitate communication within the group it is important to be alert for other factors that can block effective communication:

- Acoustic/sonic levels in room
- Seating arrangements (aim for circle or horseshoe; avoid rows/lines; consider effect of type of seating – hard, soft)
- Ventilation and temperature
- Quality of lighting and mood induced
- Time of day (after lunch/before breaks/morning/evening)
- Proximity of other groups, activities

Once you are aware of these physical factors you can alter them or in some way compensate for them.

Exchanging information

An important part of communicating effectively and functioning smoothly as a team is people's ability to exchange information relevant to the task or issue under consideration. Failure to do so can cause anger, resentment, and separation among members and impair the work of the group.

Very often a group has the information it needs to solve a problem or make a plan of action, but is unable or unaware of how to retrieve the data and put it together in such a way that an accurate or creative solution emerges. I find it valuable with most groups at this stage to spend time looking at ways of encouraging members to be assertive and energetic in eliciting and contributing information and knowledge about given problems and situations.

Exercises can again be helpful in creating positive experiences of information exchange and Chapter 10 gives examples of exercises that I have found particularly useful.

Promote collaborative norms and values

I said earlier that the group should have appropriate norms and values which encourage and support the use of the various skills involved in working together. You can do this by reinforcing such norms and values as they appear through praise, acknowledgement, and approval. Alternatively, you can actively intervene in particular ways to promote certain values and attitudes.

Encourage mutual relationships

If someone reveals a problem or difficulty, ask other people if they share some aspect of this problem. Do not jump in immediately to resolve the problem. Let the problem become a group theme for a while and encourage people to talk about it from different personal angles.

Make confrontation a communal affair

Occasionally you may have to challenge or confront someone in the group. On another occasion it may well be that you draw attention to some of the unspoken or silent rules that operate in groups and make them less than they could be. Try to avoid this appearing as a personal attack on your part:

> I'd like to tell you about something I've noticed.

Point out the implications of the incident for everyone in the group:

> Because I believe it has a great deal to say to each of us about the way we work together.

Present it as an opportunity to develop more awareness or try out new behaviours:

> Perhaps there is something that we have been missing or need to change.

Invite members to explore it collectively:

> Could we take a look at it?

In this way challenge and confrontation become a productive and normal part of group life and something that every member has an investment in.

Promote dialogue instead of monologue

Try to prevent yourself or group members making speeches and sermons. Encourage the art of short delivery. Get into the way of asking for feedback: 'What do you think?', 'Would anyone like to comment on this?', 'How do other people feel about this?' If people do go on, do not be afraid to interrupt and point out what is happening in the group or what it is like for you to experience this monologue.

Look for any opportunity which will allow you to initiate conversation and draw in as many people and viewpoints as possible.

Insist on acceptance and respect between members

Frequently members disregard, dismiss, or undervalue each other's contributions and communications and this can cause bitterness, feelings of inferiority, and resentment. Make it a rule that people are heard out, that a contribution is considered and even if not used, that the member is appreciated. It often happens that in a project, members with a strong interest in the task can be dismissive of others who are not as proficient but may be able to make a contribution at the emotional level to the maintenance and well-being of the group. In these instances it is important to point out the value of maintenance behaviours and demonstrate how complementary the members and their talents are. Maintenance functions are frequently ignored when a group gets absorbed in a project so it is essential to teach the group to respect its need to work on this level and value its experts in this field.

By paying attention to these necessary skills and values you can help the group get a real sense of itself as able to collaborate, exchange information, and co-ordinate its activities. In turn this improves the quality of group experience and deepens the degree of closeness with fellow members.

Guiding at the emotional level of group affection

At this stage of its development the emotional life of the group is very rich, intense, and powerful and manifests in every aspect of activity. The basic theme for the individual concerns his efforts to determine the degree of closeness he wants to give and wishes to receive from other group members. In some situations this is not always going to be what the member desires and feelings of jealousy, antagonism, resentment, and frustration are common. In other instances two or more members may form deep and intimate attachments which, while satisfying for them, can enrage the rest of the group who may feel excluded and devalued.

Throughout, the group has to face up to the rights, expectations, obligations, responsibilities, and consequences of intimacy and the deepening of feelings. Helping individuals and the group negotiate the complexities and demands of interdependence requires a sensitivity, tolerance, and compassion from the worker which I believe is in keeping with the notion of guide as it has been outlined earlier.

Legitimizing feelings

People are continually encountered in group settings who are uncomfortable with certain or all of their feelings, and their attempts to deny or block the expression of these feelings not only makes life very difficult for them but deprives the group of power, colour, and depth. These people often feel guilty or ashamed of their emotional needs and experiences and may require some extra help during this stage to open up a little more or manage feelings which are rising up within them.

It is valuable to spend some time exploring the range of emotions available to the individual and encourage people to talk openly about their experiences of anger, jealousy, attraction, and joy with each other. Frequently members will say that certain feelings are positive and others negative, or to be avoided. What I often find is that feelings which one might expect to be positive – tenderness, sympathy, affection, respect, and expressions of need and attraction to one another – are difficult for people to allow or express publicly.

It is important to remove any accompanying guilt or shame about these feelings and encourage members to express themselves more openly. Exercises will help but what I find most influential in legitimizing the expression of feeling in the group is my willingness to reveal my own feelings about members and events. I have often noticed that after I disclose feelings in the group, people seem less awkward and more spontaneous with their feelings.

So do not be afraid to lead with your own feelings in situations. Tell people about the effect the group is having on you. Discuss with members any difficulties you have in relating to them and how you feel about it. Your own relationship with the feeling function, attitudes, and behaviours concerning emotions does determine what is implicitly or explicitly communicated in the group. Members pick up quickly from you what is acceptable or not, so do try to develop both in yourself and in the group an ethic which encourages expression rather than repression of feelings.

Chapter 9 contains a section on working with feelings which contains more suggestions and practical advice. The important point to remember here, is that at the affection stage, emotional issues abound for people and you must help the group become more comfortable with its feelings since it is through the expression and acceptance of emotion that members will begin to reach out and come into contact with each other.

Sexual and romantic relationships in the group

Because of the dominance of affection and intimacy issues at this stage you may not be surprised in some groups to discover that two members have become sexually involved with each other. This can be an extremely sensitive area for all concerned and one that can appear to present worrying ethical and technical problems for you:

- Is this a matter for the couple themselves?
- Does the group have any rights or interests?
- What is private and what is communal in a group setting?
- Should you raise the issue or wait for it to emerge (if at all)?
- How do you handle such a sensitive matter?

These and a dozen other questions raise issues about privacy, responsibility, the personal, and the political, and tend to centre around the relationship of the individual to the group. They can impose severe strain on you as a worker because you need to find some way of balancing group needs and individual desires if they are not to destroy one another. Let us look at some issues which from my own experience in this area may help if you have to deal with the emergence of sexual relationships at this stage in the group.

How it is raised

I have experienced four main ways in which members' intimate relationships have come to be on the agenda of the group:

- The couple involved raised it; felt it was important to inform colleagues of their relationship because it affected their perception of and relationship with other members. They believed, rightly as it turned out, that it could affect how other members related to them.
- The relationship emerged as the causal factor when exploring presenting problems of conflict, jealousy, or resentment between some group members.
- I have on occasion, challenged when a couple's relationship was interfering with the work of the group through them splitting off in sessions.
- The group would refer to a relationship indirectly through jokes, hints, or comments but were unwilling to look at it directly. I addressed the group's difficulty in finding a way of dealing with their concerns about the relationship.

It is important to remember that the collective reality of the group is such that at some level everyone knows sooner or later what is happening between two fellow members. Unless this is acknowledged and varying viewpoints aired and explored the relationship can become a problem for the group and obliged to remain out of awareness. In some situations the cost of keeping this knowledge hidden or out of the public consciousness of the group is the diverting of a good deal of energy away from purpose and task and this can often result in suspicion, conflict, resentment, and a sense of phoniness.

Carefully watch for those openings that will permit the group to approach and explore a difficulty that everyone knows is around. My experience is that there is usually a pronounced sense of relief when we finally join forces on an issue that has not been openly faced before.

The issues involved

- *The head–heart split:* Group members may be understanding and even accepting at an intellectual level of a couple's right to pair. However, they can often experience great tension and conflict because they also have an opposite emotional reaction of resentment, jealousy, or anger. The psychic dissonance caused by contradictory feelings may be projected with great vehemence onto the couple who are blamed for being selfish and for disrupting the group.

- *Exclusivity:* The emergence of a sexual or romantic relationship creates the perception of a boundary and some degree of exclusivity around the couple whether it is wished for or not. This can generate feelings of anger and jealousy. There may be a sense that the original group has been diminished in some way; that the couple now form a separate sub-group or are no longer as available or accessible as they have been. One or more members may feel rejected and feelings of inferiority and worthlessness may be the motivating energy behind expressions of anger or jealousy.

- *Confidentiality and trust:* Particularly where relationships have a strong sexual dimension, issues of confidentiality and trust become important. There may be consequences for the couple and other members if their relationship became known outside the group and this can affect how open or defensive people are in their sharing and exploration. Similarly, the presence in the group of particular moral or religious viewpoints plays a significant role in whether and how the relationship is acknowledged and in what manner it is received.

The worker's role

The complexities of human relationships are too intricate to be dealt with as if they are simple problems with simple solutions, particularly in the area of sexuality. What you can be sure of is that you will be faced with apparently contradictory and irreconcilable demands from all sides. However, a workable approach to this kind of person versus group situation can be developed by thinking out the needs and values you are trying to meet and preserve. Some of them might be:

- The need to provide good leadership.
- The group's need to be productive.
- The needs for personal affirmation felt by each member of the group.

Extending this thinking to the couple and the group it is apparent that they also have needs and values which they are trying to meet:

- The need for affirmation of personal worth.
- The need for personal acceptance.
- The need for influence.

It is clear then that there are certain values and needs which you and each group member have a common investment in meeting and maintaining. What you set about doing now is converting these values into procedures for action and resolution.

In some situations it may be appropriate to talk to the couple first and obtain their permission to bring up their relationship and the relevant issues in the group since it does involve everybody. Talk about the values you hold for the group and about the values that are important for them. Try to create some sense of the relationship between the couple and the group and their reciprocal responsibilities. Note any conflicts or differences between you that could be amplified negatively in the group. If the couple are unwilling to bring it up do not insist. A situation will invariably arise which involves members' emotional reactions to the pair and this may offer a more appropriate opportunity to look at what is involved.

When and if the matter is brought to the group try to work on the assumption that there are shared concerns and mutual needs which if explored sensitively and thoroughly, can benefit everyone. Help and allow members to express their thoughts and feelings and look for opportunities to bring out the underlying issues. Challenge attempts by the group to avoid or deal covertly with issues as this will only increase suspicion and distrust. Above all, do not look for or accept instant resolution. The struggles with intimacy and sexuality may bring to the surface very real and painful conflicts for the men and women in your group which in the end may have to be lived with rather than resolved.

Foster goodwill

It is my experience that there exists in the group, and particularly at this stage, an impulse to manifest goodwill. By this I mean that members exhibit spontaneous altruistic and selfless tendencies. Members will show compassion for each other, behave generously, and act in a way which demonstrates awareness of their interconnectedness. They may also show awareness of and concern about social, political, and international issues and connect them with events in their own group life. A discussion about the need to keep the group room tidy can lead to indignation being expressed at environmental pollution; consideration of alternatives to exploitive behaviour in the group can give way to revulsion with wars, racism, sexism, and prejudice in society.

If this impulse is not tapped or is in some way repressed, group members can experience feelings of impotence, powerlessness, and shame: 'We should be doing more', 'It's too far gone', 'What's the point?', 'I can't do anything about it'. Cynicism and frustration can become a way of life in the group. The impulse towards goodwill is a very clear demonstration of the workings of the love principle and it is important to find ways of expressing this in action.

It can be helpful to encourage your group to meet with other groups through sports competition (although be careful the competitive element doesn't take over), hosting visits, sharing residential experiences, or joint work on a project. Your group might also be interested in working with handicapped or underprivileged groups in the community – children, elderly, prisoners' wives, and the like. Projects to clean up the neighbourhood, collect money for famine victims, or assist in funding a kidney dialysis machine at the local hospital may provide other ways in which the group can express its goodwill, develop a healthy idealism, and engage in compassionate service.

When these impulses towards goodwill emerge, do not receive or dismiss them immediately as avoidance techniques. You must not ignore the necessity of working with group members on legitimate concerns. It is quite natural that as the group becomes more caring and compassionate of itself members become more aware of the pain and crisis around them and move to do something about it. You have a responsibility to guide the group to express their concern in a realistic and enthusiastic manner.

Guiding at the intellectual level of group affection

At this stage of group development you can see the emergence of a clearer direction and firm plans to carry out group goals. It is important that you guide the group by:

- Praising members' ability to think creatively.
- Reinforcing their ideas.
- Encouraging members to apply their ideas.
- Creating opportunities for members to take responsibility for their plans and ideas.

Encourage choice

Members will experience the group as satisfying and assume a greater degree of responsibility for tasks and projects if they feel that they can exercise real choice about the options available. Making any choice is a risky business for many people and it is sometimes easier to go along with the ideas of others. One of my tasks at this stage is to develop in the individual and the group the ability to be responsible and to freely choose a particular course of action. This means that I continually look for opportunities in which members can experience themselves initiating action rather than reacting or submitting to an event. At the simplest level encouraging someone to express their thoughts and feelings about an incident provides them with the opportunity to assert themselves in relation to the situation. Even if this does not automatically result in the situation changing it can create awareness for the person that he has his own ideas and has the power to affirm and assert them.

I encourage members to see themselves as involved in an on-going process of making choices and discerning between options about themselves and each other.

Let me give an example of a favourite method of exploring and developing the idea of choice and self-responsibility in the group. At a suitable time I select an incident or event which is emotionally alive for group members. I then ask the members to form themselves into a living sculpture or a still photograph, in a way which symbolizes the conflicts and issues involved. In turn I ask each group member such questions as:

- What are you feeling/thinking now?
- What do you want to do?
- What do you need in this situation?
- What do you see happening now?
- What would you like to happen?
- What do you think would happen if . . .?
- What are the possibilities in this situation for you?
- What are you afraid of/avoiding?
- Is there anything else you could do?
- What choice could you make if this should occur again?

These questions reveal the underlying feelings and themes in the critical incident and give a fuller picture of what is going on. They also open up the possibility that the situation can be changed and that people can choose alternative behaviours. It can be interesting to repeat the sculpture or photograph to show the transformation brought about by awareness of choice potentials.

As far as possible I try to make my interventions capitalize upon, and enhance whatever choosing capacity exists in the person or situation. This can lead to more mature self-assertion, willingness to risk, and an openness in acknowledging mistakes or the need for help. Invariably this results in more honest and smoother relationships. So do try where possible, to devolve as many choice-making opportunities onto individuals and the group as you can. By increasing the number of choices which the group and its members have to make, you encourage cohesion, collaboration, maturity, and self-esteem.

Foster creativity

There are many occasions when a group considering a problem or an aspect of a project reaches an impasse and is unable to go any further. This can cause frustration, tension, or discomfort due to the failure to produce an adequate solution and members may become disheartened and even give up. It is important that there is a tradition within the group which supports the view that the problem is a challenge and invitation to be creative and that with time and effort a constructive solution can be found.

You can promote such a tradition by inculcating values and norms which encourage critical thinking and questioning, reformulation, originality, and innovation. The development of this type of value can be facilitated by practice and training in creative thinking, so do consider devoting a portion of time in some of your sessions to training members to seek out alternative perspectives, reformulate problems, and develop their imagination and intuitive ability. Brainstorming, for example, is one short but powerful procedure for encouraging divergent or creative thinking while involving every member. The next three chapters contain ideas and exercises which I have found valuable in my own practice and which I am sure will help you improve the creative quality and productivity of your own group.

Review

- The affection stage of the group is analogous to maturity.
- Members explore opportunities for intimacy and interdependence.
- The worker plays a less central role. The metaphor of the guide is useful as a way of encouraging the group to do more of its own work.
- The worker engages in a series of tasks with the group in order to develop teamwork and foster intimacy, goodwill, creativity, and choice.

Chapter 7

Work at the ending stage of the group: separation issues

The date of ending for some groups is determined at the outset. The number of sessions or the length of time that the group will run for is established before the group begins. In other groups termination is expected to occur upon completion of a particular task or whenever it is decided that members have achieved their goals and objectives.

However, there are other situations where a group does not coalesce; there is a heavy loss or turnover of members; workers may leave the group and termination can occur. I am not referring to these instances when I discuss ending of the group in this section. I want to look at the natural and planned termination of the group and the separation issues that are part of this stage.

The approach of termination is a psychic shock which group members react to according to their preferred method of coping with anxiety. The group is finishing and the basic issue for members is how to handle separation with least personal discomfort. Members look for ways of avoiding or denying the reality that their group is to end and when this fails to work may regress to previous states of group disorganization.

At the same time that members are trying to avoid the ending of the group there is a growing acknowledgement of the finality of termination and a willingness to face and accomplish it. However, right up until the final moment there may well be a strong tension between these two desires that can manifest in a wide variety of confused and contradictory behaviour.

There are a number of themes to look out for in the final stages:

- *Denial*: Members may express surprise or claim to have forgotten that the group would end. Members may plan to continue on their own after the formal ending or look towards reunions.

- *Regression*: This involves a sliding back into earlier group experiences and relationship patterns accompanied by increased dependence on the worker. Attempts may be made to reactivate the problems or needs that led to the group being set up originally.
- *Flight*: Destructive and aggressive behaviour may be directed towards each other, the worker, equipment, and activity. People drop out early or join other groups.
- *Reviewing*: This involves going over group experiences and reminiscing about past events and memories. It can be integrative in that it is an attempt to evaluate the meeting of the group experience and prepare members for letting go of each other.

These themes generate ambivalent behaviours and feelings which are confusions and distortions of the love and will energies (see page 147).

In general, I find that the longer members have been together the more visible and pronounced is their anger and mourning of the passing of the group. A group which has been meeting weekly for nine months will experience themselves as losing more than a group which has met for six sessions. The shorter group, however, will still experience a scaled-down version of what occurs in its older relative if it has at all bonded. So whether your group lasts for a day, six sessions, or nine months you can expect to find some of these manifestations of grief and anger at separation.

Let us look at the role of the worker in this final stage.

Working with the group at termination

As groups move towards their conclusion the worker again becomes a central figure and his major task is to help the members let go of the group and move away. As we have seen, this is an emotionally distressing time for members and can make huge demands on the worker who in all probability is trying to deal with his own separation issues.

I find that members look to me to be group mother, father, and guide all at the same time: because of their anxiety and distress they need nurturing but they also need reminding that there are clear boundaries and limits. At other times, members are well able to contain their feelings and review their work with little need of my intervention.

Manifestations of ending and separation

- Denial that the group is ending
- Delaying or prolonging work
- Frenzied work activity
- Rejection of work
- Sabotage and destruction of programme and materials
- Clinging together for comfort
- Reduced interaction and involvement
- Absenteeism
- Lateness
- Premature endings
- Abdication of responsibility
- Overdependence on worker
- Rejection, provoking, challenging of worker
- Rejection, anger, challenging of other members
- Blaming, scapegoating, finding fault
- Irruption of unresolved incidents
- Feelings of guilt, shame about levels of contribution
- Depression, despair, anxiety, grief
- Feelings of loss and abandonment
- Planned reunions

Underlying needs and motives

- To avoid separation
- To maintain group experience
- To begin again
- To deal with painful feelings
- To punish worker and 'bad' members
- To destroy group

Here are some suggestions that might help you work with your group at this stage.

Working with the group at the physical level of separation

Members' interest and investment in the group is beginning to wane and your main job now is to emphasize movement away from the group and towards other groups, members' own community, or workplace.

Complete group tasks

Aim to complete and resolve any remaining tasks left to the group and draw attention to any delaying or prolonging activity. Be alert for any over-enthusiastic approach to work which might suggest a desire to deny or preclude the group ending. I find it important to be visible with my expectation that members will complete individual tasks and join with me in concluding group projects. This seems to make ending less threatening and more in the nature of a normal passage or development.

Permit activity to become less rewarding

There is a thin line between allowing activity to become less attractive and rewarding and letting your programme collapse into boredom and monotony, which increases the risk of precipitating early withdrawal by members. What you should aim at is a gradual reduction in attraction and interest in activity, as a way of increasing members' motivation to conclude the business of separation and look outside the group for new and more stimulating relationships and experiences.

To encourage this, avoid any activity which challenges the group to further accomplishments such as competition or new projects. Activity which is stimulating, exciting, gives high rewards, or encourages a lot of group interaction should also be avoided. If you find that members are complaining of boredom you may have made activity too bland and it would be important to reintroduce some favoured activity if you are not to force members to leave prematurely. However, complaints about boredom may also reflect resistance and anger about the impending termination. In other instances I have found that the group has naturally come to an end and attempting to continue until the official end is uncreative and tedious.

In some groups you can facilitate the idea of moving out by arranging visits outside the group which prepare members for transition into workplace, community, school, or college. Visitors or guest speakers may be invited into the group to help members with enquiries about welfare rights, accommodation needs, and other points relating to life apart from the group.

Encourage ritual and celebration

I am always surprised at the attitude of those groupwork teachers and practitioners who view the farewell party as contrived, false, and beneath the dignity of the worker. By encouraging group workers to see the farewell party as an immature attempt to deny or sublimate the end of the group I believe we miss something important and deep in human experience.

The ending of the group is a kind of death and will be experienced by many members as the passing of a particular time in their lives. They need to mark this passing in a way which celebrates the importance of the experience in their lives and gives a sense of completion. At the same time they are aware that with the ending of the group there comes opportunity for new relationships and experiences and the invitation to transfer the growth and learning that took place in the group.

All cultures have recognized the pain and celebration, the death and transformation inherent in times of transition and have marked these occasions with a rite of passage – birth, death, initiation and marriage ceremonies and rituals. Similarly the ending of the group is an experience of separation and initiation, finishing and beginning which can speak to something real and deep in us. I believe it demands and warrants its own rite of passage. Obviously this will vary according to the purpose for which the group met, the time spent together, intimacy generated, and so on. It can vary from a party for members in the last session to a drink in the pub or a meal together after the last session. The important point is that you should create an end for the group which celebrates, synthesizes, and symbolizes for members what the group was all about.

If you want to be more prosaic about the ending of the group you can see the ending ritual as a way of helping the group to relax and wind down. Many groups are very task-oriented and minimize or forget the need to slow down, rest, and take pleasure in their labour. Marking the end of the group in the ways I have suggested brings home to members the necessity of maintenance activities and provides an opportunity for informality, fun, and saying goodbye.

Working with the group at the emotional level of separation

As soon as people know that the ending of the group is really going to come they deal with this knowledge by using strategies that often come from earlier in their lives. This can cause a great deal of emotional disruption among members depending on the purpose and intimacy of the group. Here are some ideas to help you to work with the feelings and emotions that are prevalent at this time.

Sort out your own feelings

The first thing to be aware of is that you have been very closely involved in the life of the group. You have been a part of the conflict, the resolutions, and the decisions that were made. The group has been a satisfying, frustrating, exciting, boring, painful, and happy experience for you. You have nurtured members through the difficult and awkward stages of their life, provided them with stability and boundary when they were in open revolt against your leadership, and you have had to sit back and let them learn through their own efforts when you could have done it faster! The point is this – the group is also ending for you and you have your own feelings and thoughts about this.

You may be glad, sad, or a mixture of both and so it is important to spend time preferably with a supervisor or colleague, looking at your own feelings about the group ending. Being clear about how the ending affects you, ensures that you do not get swamped or overwhelmed by members' feelings and are free to support the group at this difficult time. Acknowledging feelings of sadness or loss, to yourself first of all, enables you subsequently to be visible with them in the group and model for members a more appropriate way of being in relationship with their own feelings. It also helps you identify the emotional themes that are likely to be around in the group and develop strategies for highlighting and facilitating them.

Deal with separation anxieties

Give members permission to have feelings about the end of the group and encourage them to share these collectively. I try to give some structure to this by building in small sessions where members can talk about what they appreciated in the group and what they resented. This has the effect of bringing feelings to the surface, balancing them, and channelling them effectively.

View expressions of guilt, failure, and incompetence as signs of sadness or repressed anger and do not allow them to be put forward as reasons for the group ending. Allow appropriate levels of grief and anger to be expressed while maintaining boundary and avoid being hooked into punitive behaviour or made to reject members. I find the simplest way of working with such behaviour is to describe what is happening and wonder aloud what is behind it. Members are usually able to verbalize and reflect on their motives quite quickly.

Members may need help to complete unfinished business with each other or find it difficult to say goodbye to each other. It can be useful to spend time in pairs doing this or you may prefer to use exercises in which everybody can participate.

What can often make ending more difficult for members is their association of group termination with other unresolved or painful life experiences of separation, loss, abandonment, and bereavement. It is not uncommon for some members to talk openly about the death of parents or relatives and bring into the group emotional material from these events. Although the ending of a group can activate very deep feelings of pain and shock you should not allow yourself to be frightened or put off by this. You can create a positive experience of termination for your group which can go a long way towards healing and redeeming past endings, and showing people that not all separations have to be brutal and bloody.

As you help people deal with their good and bad feelings you will find that they are better able to accept separation and dissolve the group. Allow this to be a difficult time for members and respond to them with compassion, understanding, and acceptance.

Working with the group at the intellectual level of separation

It is important to help members conceptualize what the group experience has meant to them and be clear about what they are taking away from the group. A major activity at this stage is to create time and space where members can evaluate their involvement and progress. This is a different procedure from the reminiscing type of review that members typically engage in. Evaluation is a structured part of the group's work and has clear objectives:

- To determine the value of the group to the individual.
- To gauge progress in achieving individual goals.
- To assess whether group objectives were achieved.
- To determine what aspects of the group require modification.

The particular purpose of your group will determine what you evaluate for and how you conduct this. I have a particular format that I use in most groups because I find it a simple but powerful way of generating meaning, making connections, and focusing members on their future outside the group. Depending on the type of group I am working with I will ask members to write or draw in response to my questions. I preface the evaluation by repeating familiar themes to my group members – the idea of journey, of unfolding, and of process.

Where have you come from?

What were your goals/objectives at the start of the group? What were your hopes/ambitions/fears/anxieties? What was the group like for you? What were the times of joy/pain/highs/lows? What did you enjoy/regret, appreciate/resent?

Where are you at now?

What have you achieved/changed/learned? Are you satisfied/frustrated with what you have accomplished? What comments can you make about yourself now? What would you change/modify about the group/programme/sessions?

Where are you going to in your life?

What is the direction you wish to go in? What do you need to do in your life? What is your next step/goal/possibility? What do you still need to change/achieve/learn?

What is in your way?

What prevents you from changing/achieving/learning? What blocks you from going in this direction? What are you avoiding/overlooking/refusing?

What will help you?

What do you need to help you change/learn? What do you need to develop in yourself? What skills/qualities/knowledge do you need? Where will you get them from?

These five headings provide a framework for members which begins to help them understand their experience in the group and creates context, orientation, and perspective so that the group is not perceived as an isolated event but is woven into their lives.

Encourage people to reflect and abstract what learning and growth took place; what personal and interpersonal skills they acquired. This will help individuals view their membership in a more objective light and lessen feelings of grief or sadness by showing how personally beneficial involvement in the group was.

You may wish to spend time helping the group plan more specific follow-up needs. This may require you to be available to offer help after the group terminates or may take the form of a 'reunion' to gauge 'success' on a longer timescale. Be careful that follow-up is seen for what it is and not used as an attempt to continue or prolong the group.

The experience of leaving the group is not an easy one for either the members or the leader so make plenty of time available for the group to work through the separation. Don't avoid or skimp on this stage of the group's life, because if handled well the experience of ending, despite feelings of sadness and grief, can foster personal satisfaction and self-reliance, with members leaving the group feeling that they can make it on their own.

Review

- The separation stage of the group is analogous to death and brings up issues to do with ending, termination.
- Members can experience this as a time of great anxiety.

- The worker is more dominant in this stage and may intervene as group mother, father, and guide, as appropriate.
- The worker helps members to deal with feelings about ending, to review involvement, and to separate.

Chapter 8

The foundations of creative groupwork

The practice of groupwork involves a dialectical and syncretizing process and the group worker if he is to be in any way creative, is required to embrace and reconcile a number of contradictions and opposing truths. Indeed the power and efficacy of the medium is a function of the degree to which a worker can creatively transcend two apparent paradoxes. These paradoxes can be stated in the form of assertions which I believe represent four cornerstones of groupwork practice.

- Groupwork is a rational activity.
- Groupwork is an intuitive and spontaneous activity.

- The group worker is separate, non-directive, value-free.
- The group worker is involved, sympathetic, and committed.

Any one of these statements can be acknowledged as 'true' by a group worker who may then proceed to construct a philosophy and operate on the basis of his truth. I have done it myself with each of these statements, at different stages in my career. Increasingly, however, I have found that my practice is enhanced by affirming the presence and validity of all four statements on all occasions.

The process of moving to this position has been somewhat like allowing oneself to be, first, influenced by one ideology and then to allow experience to challenge and shatter it, and finally to transcend the contradictions in a synthesis which unfolds through a new commitment to more comprehensive goals. The experience is confusing and painful and there is a tendency to avoid or minimize frustration and stop the process by adopting one particular party line: groupwork is either rational or it is not; the worker is either non-directive or he influences the group explicitly.

I believe the truth is nearer to a position which is inclusive of the potentials and properties of each of these perspectives. Creative groupwork is able to reconcile apparent opposites and see the complementarity in contradiction. Unfortunately there is a tendency on the part of many beginning group workers to slip into a rational, technical style of intervention which can limit the worker's capacity for relevant response and dialogue and confuses means with ends. In order to redress the balance and show the importance of a supra-rational approach to working with people, the remainder of this chapter is devoted to considering and rehabilitating the more experiential aspects of the foundational groupwork paradoxes.

Groupwork as art, faith, and science

I am convinced that working with a group is more of a synthesis between art and faith than the logically evolved and dispassionate procedure that some applied social scientists would have us believe. While it is clearly essential to have a body of theoretical concepts and technique, I would suggest that groupwork is more than the 'appliance of science', and needs to include and express those other dimensions of human experience.

If it is to be a powerful and humane medium, groupwork requires:

- That the worker intervene at least as stylistically as the artist who bases his work on intuitive, affective, and aesthetic judgements.
- That the worker function out of a deep conviction and vision of the wholeness, creativity, and possibility inherent in the group, which matches the faith of the believer who knows what is and what can be.

I am encouraged in these views by recent research from the field of group therapy which explores the various factors and processes contributing to improvement in the patient's condition.[1] Probably the most famous work was carried out by Irvin Yalom who in 1970 identified twelve 'curative factors'.[2] Some of the more important of these curative or therapeutic factors are:

- *Self-understanding.*
- *Interaction.*
- *Universality*: member's realization that his problems are not unique.
- *Instillation of hope*: belief that participation in the group will be beneficial.
- *Altruism*: benefit derived from recognition that group members can help each other.
- *Guidance* ⎤
- *Indentification* ⎦ worker's influence.
- *Cohesiveness*: the degree to which each member feels accepted and valued.
- An *'existential' factor*: being authentic, taking responsibility for self.

I have worked in a wide variety of group settings and it is my experience that these curative factors apply not only in therapy groups but contribute greatly to the well-being and productivity of most, if not all, group situations. I believe they reveal the existence in groupwork of deep taproots into the realms of art and faith and clearly make the point that working with a group is about the creation of a fellowship bond in which the worker cannot avoid being other than an active and influential moral agent.

The discovery of these therapeutic factors seems to me to devolve a special responsibility onto the worker to create just those conditions in the group which will foster awareness, perception, and belief among members and help them achieve their goals. To do this the worker must not only intervene in an aesthetic way but he must also have clear beliefs about the value and importance of what he is doing.

If he is to work imaginatively and sympathetically with people and bring a quality of presence to the group which is spontaneous, genuine, and enabling, the worker must aim to synthesize in his practice many different aspects of the human experience. This is very much a personal and ongoing part of being a group worker and not one that can be taught. However, it can be encouraged and developed and we will now consider some of the basic values, resources, and attitudes that will help you become a more effective and creative influence in the group.

The importance of values and vision in groupwork

These therapeutic factors that we have been looking at really seem to revolve around possibilities in the group setting which are considered desirable. However, while one might desire to include in one's group design variables such as the existential factor or altruism, their inclusion is not something which can be very easily planned or replicated in any setting. If we are to have any regular access to these processes, a shift in perception is required from a mechanistic view to one which allows that groupwork is more than a rational activity and that in its 'irrationality' is revealed a deep affinity with the spontaneity and sympathy encountered in painting, poetry, or music. And at the heart of groupwork, as at the core of these supra-rational activities, is a concern with the transmission of values and the incarnation of a vision.

Values are really what are most important to people and will exert influence on group members to act in their direction.

Values motivate behaviour and give us a general direction to move in. They provide a vision of what is possible; of what we may be. If you have what appears to be an intractable problem, participation in a carefully constructed group experience with its promise of support, care, and opportunities to learn, can provide you with the hope that things may be different and stimulate more creative coping and management behaviours. Frequently the major inducement which a group can offer its members is the opportunity to select and engage with values which will assist and motivate them to change.

This is important news for the group worker. Values create vision and vision creates goals. Our work can only be as effective as the vision and range of possibilities that we hold out to group members. Without a sense of what we may be – a goal to aim towards – members can have no hope; they experience no enthusiasm. So it is incumbent upon the group worker to be clear and thoughtful about the values the group strives to generate and the vision of possibility he wishes to manifest for members, until such time as they can see clearly for themselves.

For some of you this may appear patronizing and even interfering. Frequently I come across an attitude amongst group workers which asserts that it is essential to be value-free or at the least neutral. The group worker is one who believes in the client's right to self-determination; does not make value judgements and would never seek to impose upon group members. That such an attitude is in itself a value judgement seems to escape its adherents.

With a little thought it is evident that this particular attitude is neither realistic nor desirable. While in no way wishing to compromise the integrity of another person it should be obvious that it is not possible for a worker to eliminate the impact of his own values.

There is simply no situation in a group which does not imply choice at some level of consciousness or suggest that one action has been selected or preferred as more desirable than another. Intervening to protect, support, or challenge a group member, for example, all indicate that a worker regards this activity as having some advantage or value. Another problem I find with the value-free perspective is that it fails to understand that values are essentially self-determined. It is extremely difficult to change another person's value system. Value change will only truly come about when it makes sense to the person concerned. Victor Frankl writing about his experiences in a Nazi concentration camp clearly makes the point that a person's values and the internal choices that related to them could still flourish amidst the most savage oppression and duress.[3]

By now it should be clear that I see the group worker as a 'carrier of values', to quote Alan Klein and like him I see the most important aspect of the worker's method as the effort to help group members 'find their own values'.[4] But if you are really going to help members find their own values, it is necessary that you think long and carefully about your own, since your relationship with group members will quickly and clearly demonstrate what is actually important to you and how you see people relating to each other as human beings. Neither can you expect members to create a personal vision of what is most expressive of them until you have offered them your vision of what it could be like in this group. You cannot even really expect members to use the service offered if you are unable or unwilling to advance your vision of the possibilities and choices inherent in attending the group.

Identification with the worker is one of the primary dynamics for changes and it is inevitable that as members come to trust and like you, they will internalize aspects of your behaviour, values, and vision. You cannot avoid being a model for the people you work with nor should you try to avoid this. The most appropriate course of action is to accept with grace and thoughtfully work out a vision for the group which has as its core a desire to help people find their own way. Your values create your vision and your vision can create choices. The more choice you can create for members the more likely you are to be an effective and creative influence in the group and the more likely they are to achieve their goals.

The group worker's deadly sins

From personal experience I have discovered that certain themes recur in groupwork practice. I call these themes 'the group worker's deadly sins' as they seem to represent weaknesses which can only be overcome by diligence, hard work, and lots of self-forgiveness!

Ignorance

This is probably the most common condition of all and one that is really brought about by a lack of knowledge and understanding of the properties and qualities of the medium of groupwork. I find that many novice workers are blissfully unaware of:

- The organic and energetic nature of the group
- The dynamic tension of the love and will energies (members' urge to attach and the urge to separate)
- The relationships between content and process interaction, task and maintenance behaviours
- The need to include and work at the process and mainten-ance levels in a group
- The typical stages of development that a group goes through
- How to match their style of leading to the group's needs at different stages of development

Typically this results in:

- Behaviour being seen at an individual level rather than in terms of group process
- Failure to recognize the need motivating the behaviour
- Failure to intervene appropriately
- Loss of creativity, productivity; anger, resentment, frustra-tion, withdrawal
- The other deadly sins

This is an example of the importance of the rational side of working with groups. Without access to the theoretical and intellectual knowledge many group workers stumble around not knowing what to look for, influence, or co-operate with. Once they become conscious of the nature, properties, and characteristic of groups most workers find that they are more spontaneous, perceptive and skilful in their practice. The earlier chapters in this book provide helpful summaries of the main points you need to be aware of when working with a group and also contain practical suggestions.

The need to control the group

The most common practice weakness is the worker's attempt to overly control the group. This is based on two main fantasies:

- The controller is afraid of the group. If asked to reveal his worst fear, it is that the group will suddenly fly out of his control. His unconscious fantasy is that the darker side of human nature will escape in the group, overwhelm him, and cause others to act in a destructive way. He is frightened by the number of people in the group, feels alone, and threatened by the spontaneity and unpredictability of group members. So he tries to programme people and events in order to avoid the imminent chaos. Needless to say, that stage of the group's life which is naturally more provocative is a nightmare for him.
- Another type of controller appears to believe that he is responsible for the group and so must do whatever is necessary to ensure that the group is successful, well-attended, and orderly. Frequently this worker is afraid of being blamed if the group does not work out in some way and so he must exercise constant vigilance in order to avert failure. In other cases the worker reveals an unconscious contempt for group members since he is unable to allow them to be autonomous and self-determining but must continually chivvy them in the desired direction like some nineteenth-century missionary or imperialist among the colonial natives.

The controlling worker is usually not very experienced with groups or may have been a participant in a destructive and unhealthy group and his inappropriate parental and controlling behaviour is a way of maintaining order in the face of potential chaos. Unfortunately this rigid stance often energizes the rebellious adolescent in group members. Most people resent inappropriate control and will react to it in various ways. If this expression is not permitted or its form is unhealthy and immature, a negative spiral of repression and revolt, oppression and sabotage, can ensue with disastrous consequences for worker and members.

It is essential that you work out carefully your attitudes to control, discipline, and authority, preferably in the planning stage of the group – and with a colleague or supervisor – if you are going to be able to 'let go' in the group. You will need to think very seriously about the nature of responsibility. Obviously you have a responsibility to guide, protect, and facilitate the group members but equally they have responsibilities to you and to each other. Members must be expected, and allowed, to be responsible!

The particular purpose for which your group was set up and the nature of membership should largely determine the control levels in the group. If you become aware that you are having to discipline, organize, or control more than before, ask yourself:

- What is going on in this group?
- What does the individual/group need?
- What are they trying to say to me?
- Are the group goals clear, agreed, realistic?
- Are members fearful, unwilling to focus on goals?
- Are members inviting direction for some other reason?
- How do I feel about group members now?
- What am I avoiding?
- What do I need now?
- What is the best way of getting the group to work with me on this control issue?

As far as possible try to:

> * Create a situation where people are not afraid to express themselves
> * Expect members to be responsible
> * Listen carefully in order to find out what people need
> * Find and use a common language
> * Find any common ground/values between you
> * Do something together about the control problem rather than you acting alone

Fear of failure: addiction to perfection

When I first started working with groups I had a strong desire to be a good group worker. I wanted very much to be successful. Success to me meant sessions in which I intervened with perceptive and sparkling interpretations, members resolved their problems, got a lot from the group, and wanted to come back. To ensure such success, I meticulously planned each session. I worked out my objectives, selected the best exercises with care and considered in great detail, the most suitable interventions to make if this happened or that happened. Looking back I see now that my overplanning resulted in a rigid, staccato, formal style which could not cope with spontaneous or unpredictable events.

And sure enough one day in a session a young girl disclosed some detail about herself that I just could not relate to. I did not know what to say or do. The copious session notes on my knee offered no appropriate intervention. After what seemed an eternity, I blurted out that I just did not know what to do. To my amazement the other girls in the group came in immediately and affirmed and supported the girl in a very caring and down-to-earth way. I realized that my compulsive attention to detail and preoccupation with getting it right was creating in me a very arid, unimaginative, and unfeeling way of working. I was fast becoming a technician, a mechanotherapist.

The drive to be a successful group worker and my need to get things right, was masking my fear of failure. I was afraid of being a failure as a worker, looking as if I did not know what I was doing; making mistakes. I wanted to impress, to be liked, to achieve, and above all not to fail. This had resulted in overplanning and a loss of creativity and empathy. It was a revelation to me that my fear of failure and pursuit of perfection was actually slowing up progress in the group, lessening cohesion, and undermining any attempts to co-operate or collaborate. From then on I began to teach myself different attitudes and develop other ways of being in a group.

Much later as a trainer, I found that fear or shame about failure and the subsequent addiction to perfection, lay at the root of a lot of the novice group worker's activity:

- Overplanning, perfectionism, fussiness
- Working at a content level
- Avoidance of process work on feelings, atmosphere, etc.
- Self-defeating behaviour – not beginning or completing projects, delays, cancellations
- Excessive intervention
- Preoccupation with technology – video, two-way mirrors, etc.
- Desire for co-workers
- Anxiety reflected in constant course attendance, acquisition of ideas, techniques, 'skills'

On page 165 you will find some suggestions which can be useful in lessening the fear of failure in the group setting.

Comparison

I remember working with a group of teachers on ways in which they could be more creative and informal in the classroom setting. After a time I became aware of a sullenness and lack of response from them. When I challenged this and asked them to look at what was happening, it soon became clear that the teachers were comparing their own work situation with thirty 'unwilling' students in classroom conditions to the current setting where I was working with a polite, 'willing' group of adults. They were comparing their own fears, anxieties, and clumsy efforts in the class with my apparently confident and proficient approach to them. These comparisons resulted in feelings of inadequacy, lack of competence, powerlessness, and helplessness which were then projected onto me in the form of anger and resentment.

Since then I have observed on many occasions how a group

- You are not responsible for providing right answers or even any answers to problems
- Avoid being cast in the role of expert
- Insist on a communal approach to work, teambuilding, problem solving
- Develop and encourage values and norms which emphasize and allow the creative and positive aspects of failure, risk-taking, decision making, spontaneity and intuition, compassion, forgiveness
- Believe in and cultivate a collective or group wisdom which can be called on
- See the work of the individual or group as an ongoing process rather than a static project. Work more with process levels of experience
- Explore members' experiences of failure and identify favourite ways of avoiding coping, hiding. Identify idealized self-images, parental and self-expectations that contribute to a fear of failure or preoccupation with success
- Do not hide your mistakes in the group. Use them as an opportunity to model new behaviours and develop suitable norms

worker may compare himself to his co-worker or another colleague. Sometimes the comparison is with a mental picture of how the 'ideal group worker' – a composite of experience, reading, fantasy, and wish – would behave in a certain situation. The consequence of such comparisons is usually the same as it was for those teachers. Workers find themselves resentful and jealous of a co-worker or team member. They feel inadequate, deficient, and may begin to compete, try to impress or dominate. In some instances workers may render themselves impotent or powerless in the group because they cannot see how they could work like 'Dr Jack' or Carl Rogers.

One of the disturbing things about these negative comparisons is that the group worker is often unable to become involved with members because he is convinced that another person would be more effective in his group. The negative comparison activates deep-seated feelings of unworthiness and inadequacy and can create self-fulfilling patterns in the group, resulting in unhappy and frustrating experiences for everyone. If you observe in yourself or in your co-worker:

- Sudden criticism and signs of intolerance
- Rivalry, competition, need to win, achieve, impress
- Withdrawal, depression, loss of interest
- Evidence of feelings of inadequacy, incompetence, worthlessness, inferiority, jealousy
- Panic, helplessness, impotence, powerlessness
- Obsessive behaviour
- Anger, resentment, hostility
- Sudden interest in acquiring skills, attending courses

it could be that this type of comparison and self-depreciation is happening. It is vital between co-workers that this is acknowledged openly and dealt with. This may mean having to involve a third and neutral party. Similarly if you find that some of your behaviour in the group is motivated by jealousy of 'what the previous worker did', or other comparisons, it is important that you pay close attention to this if you are not to be overwhelmed and de-skilled. Talking with your supervisor or another worker can help a great deal. Disclosing some of your feelings in the group can also yield surprising insights and discoveries. As soon as you recognize the presence of a tendency to compare yourself or your group with another setting, act quickly to deal with it because these comparisons can distort reality very easily and release negative energies in the group.

Attachment to the past

A variation of the last two practice 'sins', attachment to the past, manifests in workers and members, as a yearning back to an enjoyable session, activity, or group. Statements or thoughts like, 'This group isn't the same any more', 'I wish the group were more like it was when . . .', indicate a turning away from what is happening here and now and an avoidance of possibly painful but necessary growth. At other times it may be evident that a worker is unable or unwilling to move forward, is stuck at a particular period of a group's growth or endeavour, and is repeating this in subsequent groups.

As soon as you become aware of this tendency in yourself or your co-worker, acknowledge it and look for someone to help you deal with it. Bring it up in supervision sessions or failing that, try as honestly as you can to identify your fears and anxieties in the situation. See the pattern as indicating the need for your practice to develop and grow. Try to get a sense of what you need to help you move on or face up to a particular issue, activity, or stage of growth in the group, and work out specific ways of changing your behaviour. It can be valuable to share your insight with the group if you feel capable of converting the issue into a group theme.

The truth about neutrality

Many group workers like to believe that they are neutral, non-directive, and value-free about the people they work with. I have already said that this latter belief is untenable without its opposite and on its own is in my experience very often the major source of difficulty in establishing effective interpersonal relations in the group and promoting healthy task and maintenance behaviour.

We have here in a very stark form one of the fundamental paradoxes of groupwork and indeed of the helping professions. In offering help to others the group worker must respect the personal integrity of members and must not impose his own personal preferences. And yet we have seen that the very effort to initiate the work with a group is laden with beliefs about its value, power, and efficacy otherwise it could not be offered or accepted. The worker's relationship with members is a major instrument for promoting change and it is clear that absolute neutrality would manifest as indifference which could only alienate members and at best make the experience a bland and superficial one.

The way in which I try to resolve this paradox is to make it a central feature of what the group has to offer members. I am clear and explicit about my vision of the range of possibilities inherent in the group experience and of the value of this, but I will not impose this vision on people for at its core is a belief that individuals can make choices for themselves, can determine their own reality, and must be expected to assume responsibility for this. In other words I will be involved and will actively engage with members but I will not do for them what they must do for themselves. The group represents a set of beliefs about how people can coexist together but each group and every member has to work out whether this is relevant for them and if necessary create alternatives and other ways of working. I advocate the value of mutuality and reciprocity while maintaining the individual's right to choose differently. I involve myself fully in the process while endeavouring to remain outside of it. In the next section we will explore a practice that I find crucial in helping me resolve the paradox of neutrality which exists side by side with passionate involvement.

The importance of right relations in the group

If members are to achieve personal goals and help accomplish the group task they require a healthy environment which encourages them to have intimate relationships with each other and fosters interdependence. Assagioli, who developed psychosynthesis underlines this point. He believes that 'each man may be considered as an element or a cell of a human group' and that the problems which inevitably arise can be solved by creating circumstances in which the different group members learn to work together as one.[5] In Assagioli's view these circumstances come about whenever people begin to practise 'right relations' with themselves, each other, and their environment.

Right relations is a practice which I find has exciting and powerful implications for work with groups. It includes some of the therapeutic or curative factors that we looked at earlier.

- Friendship
- Co-operation, teamwork, sharing
- Empathy
- Goodwill
- Altruism
- Sense of responsibility
- Service
- Understanding

I use right relations as a way of helping members recognize and affirm the value and uniqueness of each individual in the group; as a method of creating space in which members can learn, give, and receive, without trying to convert, convince, or impose on each other. I introduce the idea of right relations at the beginning of the group and depending on the type of membership, I may use standard trust exercises, or individuals' personal experiences to make a few simple points:

- Relationships are necessary for survival, growth, and development
- Relationship means being a part of rather than being isolated. (However, being a part of something does not mean being dependent on it.)
- Right relationship is about creating interaction and balance between people, and helping members experience the benefits of sharing and working together
- Right relations means being with other people in the way that you would wish them to be with you

In a discussion or review, conversation usually focuses around:

- What right relations means personally for members
- What would block/prevent right relations in this group
- What would facilitate right relations
- The importance of trust
- What values, norms, rules are appropriate in this group

Introducing the notion of right relations at the start of the group is more than a way of dealing with members' inclusion issues. It is the start of a practice that will influence every aspect of group functioning. The motivation which underlies the practice of right relations is one of goodwill and a desire to be in relationship with other people in a way which creates awareness, respect, and acceptance of the needs of both parties. If the group is to be a satisfying and productive experience, right relations must become the ongoing interest and concern. Certain fundamental personal and group interactive skills and values need to be encouraged.

In a group setting expression of a member's experience determines and contributes to the overall flow or process of the group. Withholding self-expression limits and starves the potential in a situation and can activate and amplify negative feelings which will disrupt right relations within the group. I try to inculcate in members an awareness of their responsibility for the quality of group experience and of their obligations to each other. I encourage members to be more visible and express what is happening for them in appropriate ways. Initially this raises issues for members about risk-taking, self-revelation, and the consequences for them and for other people. These issues have to be addressed and I find that being able to present members with a concern for right relations in the group is a useful way of providing a context or framework in which these issues can be worked through.

Frequently communications in a group are diluted or withheld because one person is unwilling to be seen to be angry or hurtful towards another, or because he is afraid of being rejected for his remarks. In these instances I encourage people to connect to their goodwill when they send and receive messages. This can often transform situations and people can give and accept feedback which they would previously have perceived as hostile or wounding. Thoughts and feelings can now be expressed as friendly information with the aim of exploring the dynamics of a situation or looking for resolution rather than seeking to obliterate the other person.

Some members can find it difficult to allow or accept the pain and distress of a colleague and will rush in to rescue the person or fix things up. In these situations I encourage the rescuer to express his own discomfort and become more aware of how efforts to help the other person are largely designed to relieve his own distress. By locating the exchange within the context of right relations it becomes possible for both the rescuing member and the distressed member to have their own reality and uniqueness without one needing to change or disallow the other. Another way in which I use and create right relations in the group is to urge members to check out their assumptions and perceptions of each other. Frequently you will see members assuming knowledge, or attributing ideas and feelings to each other which are not based on reality and which can have explosive repercussions. By checking out what they perceive or understand, with the other person's experience, members can remain in some degree of harmony and balance with each other.

Beyond these specific examples, the chief value of right relations is that it provides me with a context or holding frame within which the great paradoxes of groupwork can be contained and lived with:

- Each member is his brother's keeper and he is not
- Members are interdependent and yet autonomous
- The worker is separate and he is involved
- The worker is neutral and he is committed
- Groupwork is a rational activity and it is spontaneous

Right relations recognizes, affirms, and grows out of the essential contradiction and complementarity inherent in these antinomies. The work, values, and concerns of members, group, and worker emerge out of the tension generated by seeming opposites and the practice of right relations offers a context in which the necessity of each can be permitted and explored without one having to dismiss or obviate the other.

With practice, and continual reminder and encouragement from you, right relations can become a reality in the group, as well as a goal to aspire towards. Gradually members become more active and assertive in the group and the collective experience is healthier, deeper, and more genuine. Members come to see that there is an assured mutuality between self and other which means that the individual benefits as the group experience is enhanced.

Review

- Groupwork is an activity which arises out of the acknowledgement and synthesis of contradictions and opposing truths.
- Groupwork is a supra-rational activity which involves intuitive, subjective judgements as well as rational, technical prescriptions.
- There are a number of curative factors or values which must be present if the group is to be effective.
- Values create vision and vision creates goals.
- The group worker must be a carrier of values while aiming to help members find their own values.
- The group worker is an exemplar, model, visionary.
- There are common practice weaknesses to be recognized and overcome.
- It is important to establish right relations in the group as a practical reality, a goal/vision to aspire towards, and a context in which the paradoxes of groupwork can be reconciled.

Chapter 9

The skills of creative groupwork

Creative groupwork is a phrase that I use to describe the means by which a worker creates the psychological space necessary for the range of possibilities inherent in his vision of the group to emerge, and intervenes in a way which affirms members and facilitates the achievement of the group purpose. Here are some examples of what might be termed creative groupwork:

- Being able to work intuitively and imaginatively when familiar or traditional approaches do not seem appropriate in a situation
- Feeling comfortable working at different levels of the group experience at the same time
- Being able to work with process to help individuals or the group when stuck, flat, or tense
- Working effectively with feelings
- Using a variety of techniques to work through difficult situations in the group
- Developing the practice of right relations
- Knowing when to leave a task or programme to deal with process or maintenance issues
- Helping members articulate and work at their own operating principles rather than imposing a structure or vision upon them
- Helping members see the consequences of their behaviour, developing options, creating choice
- Encouraging the resolution of interpersonal conflict in a way which does not negate either party

If you consider this list it is clear that there are three major skills which the group worker uses to engage the group with imagination and sympathy:

- Use of self as a model or exemplar.
- Perceiving what is happening in the group and aligning with, or encouraging certain values, norms, behaviours.
- Providing structure and experiential work which will foster and train desirable behaviour and attitudes.

These skills are not new to us. In the last few chapters we have looked in detail at how you may use these practice behaviours or some combination of them in different situations. Now I want to consider them in relation to four activities that you are most likely to need to develop in your work with groups.

- Working with feelings
- Teaching members how to maintain themselves
- Teaching members how to analyse group process
- Working with difficult situations

Working with feelings

In some ways feelings are the common denominator between people in a group setting. Unconsciously each member is preoccupied with feeling states: wanting to feel happy, good, approved of, and well-regarded; feeling bad or rejected and wanting to change that. Much of the colour, diversity, and richness of group life is provided by the feeling tone of members' interactions. This is because feelings and emotions are multi-dimensional containing instinctual elements, intuition, physical and sensational experience, as well as an evaluative aspect.

Frequently members of a group may have difficulty expressing their feelings about events or situations. You can observe two main patterns.

- Members keep a tight rein on their feelings because they are afraid things will get out of control or because they see expression of feeling as weak and immature. These members do not trust feelings and try to avoid them either by consciously suppressing or unconsciously repressing them. However, unwanted feelings do not just disappear. They continue to try to enter awareness and behaviour directly or covertly and they often encounter more opposition. The result may be an unhealthy group with a flat, dead feel, or a tense, anxious group where things seem to be constantly simmering but never actually coming to the boil.

- When feelings are revealed they may be poorly or inappropriately expressed. Some members can express lots of feelings but in ways which alienate other people or disrupt group activity. One person may flare up at the least imagined slight, while another may sulk or cry at the drop of a hat.

The unhealthy thing about both of these patterns is that through a process of amplification, members can be invaded by other people's unexpressed or inappropriate feelings. This can result in a distorted perception of reality, intolerance, confusion, and hysteria. Feelings can enrich and enhance interpersonal life but all too often they disrupt it with conflict and grief. It is essential that you help members be more straightforward with their feelings if emotions are not to stand in the way of better relationships in the group. You need to teach members how to ask directly for what they want and to express appropriately what they like and dislike. Here are certain guidelines that I find useful for helping people work with feelings in the group.

Feelings are OK

In Chapter 5 I talked about legitimizing feelings and there is not much more to add. The important thing is that you help people recognize that experiencing feelings and emotions is an integral part of being human. No one has to apologize for having feelings. It is really how we act and behave around our feelings that makes them negative or positive.

Become aware of feelings

Often a group member may be unaware of what feelings he is experiencing and in some cases how to define them. It is important to draw attention to this because recognizing that he has thoughts and feelings about a situation can help an individual be less passive and more active in the group. Sometimes a simple question, 'How are you feeling right now?' is enough to evoke awareness. At other times drawing attention to visible cues and body language is valuable.

- What are you doing with your fists?
- You seem to be holding your breath
- I notice that you are drumming your fingers
- I see you're looking worried

Once a feeling has been recognized I often ask a few more questions as a way of evoking greater understanding and experience of the feeling and helping to release some of its energy.

- Where in your body do you experience this feeling?
- What does that suggest to you?
- If your feeling had a voice what would it say?
- What image does this feeling suggest?
- Can you become this image in your imagination, speak, act, behave as this image?

Accept responsibility for your own feelings

Difficult or irrational feelings do not go away by being censored or denied. They go away by being recognized, accepted, and worked through. In groups people have many different ways of not taking responsibility for their own feelings. Three of the most common are:

- Blaming others.
- Projecting onto others.
- Distancing feelings.

Frequently you will observe one member blame you or other colleagues for how they are feeling:

'If you hadn't insisted on talking about this, I wouldn't feel depressed now.'
'All this group does is talk about unhappy things. It makes me really angry.'

Usually what is happening here is that the person has been bottling up a particular feeling and the discussion has brought up emotions that he would prefer not to be aware of. It is important that you point out to the individual that such contact with someone who makes him angry or depressed is often because he is feeling this way already. Invite the person to explore what he is feeling and help him get it out of his system.

Watch out for people blaming others for what they are feeling. This often indicates a personal difficulty with a particular feeling and a need to reject or avoid it.

Try to use blaming situations to help people identify feelings that they find difficulty in expressing, as a way of improving and developing interaction in the group. Some of the more difficult feelings for people in groups are:

- Feelings of being no good/inferior/not able to do things
- Not being able to handle affection/interest from others
- Feelings of being dependent on a person/attracted/ interested in someone
- Feelings of being hurt/rejected/vulnerable/visible
- Guilt/shame
- Helplessness/powerlessness
- Being angry/wanting to punish/hurt

Another way that people in groups avoid taking responsibility for their feelings is to attribute or project onto other people qualities or emotions which in fact belong to them. Whenever I hear people making critical comments towards others I generally ask them if they can own some of the statement for themselves. In other words I ask them to consider if there is anything in their statement which could possibly apply to themselves. Very often the initial remarks can change drastically when the person takes responsibility for what he really feels instead of projecting it onto other people.

Statements like:	Can be more honestly expressed:
• You're always angry with me.	• I'm angry with you.
• You're always showing off.	• I want some attention too.
• You confuse things in the group.	• I'm jealous of the way you get what you want in the group.

People may distance their feelings by disguising them in question form: 'Does anyone feel angry about this?' usually means 'I feel angry about this'; 'I wonder if you're annoyed with me?' really means 'I feel upset/anxious/angry that you are upset/anxious/angry with me'. I strongly discourage people asking this sort of question in the group because members are seldom requesting information but really masking their own experience.

Many questions start from a hidden agenda and can be put in the form of a statement which is more explicit and less open to game playing. Another form of distancing feelings is to use 'it' or 'we' instead of 'I'. 'The group feels tense' decodes as 'I feel tense'. 'We don't seem to be in great form today' translates as 'I feel down today'.

It is important to challenge any attempt to avoid or disown feelings in the group. Firstly, because helping members own their feelings is to encourage them to be more powerful and responsible in the group. People can quickly learn to stick up for their emotional rights in the group and to be assertive without invading others or being deprived themselves. Secondly, accepting responsibility for our feelings allows the feeling to exist and therefore to change. Feelings are not static or permanent unless they are disallowed in which case they become chronic. Feelings are naturally transient, and if allowed and accepted will change appropriately. This is a prominent feature of the therapy group, where unacceptable or frightening feelings are often seen to dissipate when encountered and accepted, and a feature that I try to build in to all of the groups that I work with. Irrespective of task or purpose, people need to

recognize and take responsibility for their feelings if they are to
relate to each other honestly and create opportunities for growth
and transformation.

Exploring feelings

There is always some risk for members expressing feelings in the
group because they can never be sure how others will react. Nor can
you be sure that you will be able to facilitate the situation and
prevent it getting out of control or frightening the group. However,
if you have encouraged people to be more aware and accepting of
their feelings you have reduced much of the risk and unpredictability and members will be more likely to express their feelings in
an appropriate fashion.

One way that I encourage people to become more comfortable
with feelings is to demonstrate the importance of expressivity in
determining the quality of group experience. This fits in easily with
the ideas about right relations that we looked at earlier. I teach
members that behind every feeling, conflict, and disturbance is an
unfulfilled need that the person is trying to meet through his emotional responses and behaviour. This is not only important for the
individual but has major consequences for the group. So it is in
the group's interest to allow and respond to the feelings of its members. If the group and the person can become conscious of what is
really needed when angry, depressed, or tearful then they can
consider options and make choices to meet the need, which will
be more constructive and will enhance group and personal
experience.

I ask questions which open up these deeper needs and give me the
flexibility that is necessary to deal with feeling problems:

- What do you need right now?
- What would help you cope with this?
- Is there anything that you need from the group?
- How could things be different for you?
- What are your feelings telling you about yourself/the group?
- What are you avoiding/preventing yourself from doing?
- What are you being deprived of?
- Is there someone in the group who could help you now?

Often these sort of questions reveal the underlying need in the situation and can serve to refine and reframe the problem. It is usually not difficult to enlist the support and resource of the group to help create meaning and resolution:

- Does anyone know how John is feeling?
- Has anyone ever felt like this before?
- What was it like for you?
- What did you need?
- What were you avoiding; deprived of; being prevented from doing?
- What did you do/want to do?
- What do you think John could do?
- What would you advise John not to do?
- How do you feel about John's emotional reaction?
- What do John's feelings tell us about the group communication/trust/decision making/task/process, etc?

Sometimes penetrating to the deeper levels of a feeling reveals an emotional block which requires some release or discharge of energy. Depending on the purpose of the group, time available, and temperament of the person or couple involved you may wish to provide ways and means of expressing strong feelings. Here are some ideas taken from my work in a therapy context which I have found useful in a variety of group settings.

Stay in the here and now

If you watch people in a group you will see that they often distract themselves from uncomfortable feelings by talking about or discussing their feelings rather than experiencing them. It is important to draw attention to this and encourage members to be concrete and specific about their feeling experiences in the present tense. This simple but powerful technique creates the potential to go deeper into a feeling and co-operate with the natural impulse to discharge and complete the experience. Often this involves encouraging the person to stay with distracting feelings of frustration, being blocked, or confusion in order for the real feeling to emerge and be dissolved.

Repeat and exaggerate

Another simple technique for helping a person contact and discharge feelings is to use repetition. Sometimes a person may disclose that he is angry or sad, in a way which shows that he is inhibiting or checking the energetic aspect of the feeling. I try to identify a key phrase in the person's disclosure and ask him to repeat it several times. Usually the person is helped to contact the basic feeling and discharge it quickly. A helpful variation is to ask the person to exaggerate the phrase in some way – say it loudly, softly, shout it. Repetition and exaggeration can also be used on non-verbal language very effectively. I might ask someone to exaggerate drumming his fingers on the table to help him get in touch with some frustration or anger he is feeling. You can request a member to repeat and exaggerate any gesture, posture, behaviour, statement, or attitude.

Dialogue

Another way in which members can explore strong feelings and conflicts is to encourage them to converse with an absent person or a part of themselves which is causing distress. In the famous Gestalt empty chair technique the member imagines that the absent person or contrary part is sitting in a chair opposite and he expresses fully his feelings and all the things he is prevented from saying. This is a simple method of resolving intrapersonal and interpersonal conflicts. It can seem artificial at first but artificial does not mean false and your respect and compassion for the person will usually encourage them to get involved. A way of involving the group is to do a psychodrama where other members play different parts or people in the individual's conflict (see Chapter 10, page 206).

Physical release

Since feelings always have a physical expression, it is valuable to give practical ways of discharging feelings. Again, depending on your group, members can, among other things, do the following:

- Use a cushion to kick, punch, jump on
- Stamp on the floor
- Push against the wall
- Tear up paper
- Wring a towel (neck substitute!)
- Shout, scream
- Squeeze a tennis ball

This sort of expression of feeling need not be confined simply to therapy groups. Strong feelings arise in the work group or the classroom and being able to acknowledge them and offer an appropriate discharge is a valuable and creative service to give any group of people. These few techniques do not require a lot of knowledge or expertise and will carry you through most situations which involve feelings. All they require on your part is sensitivity and a willingness to be attentive and imaginative.

Some things to be aware of when working with feelings

- *Deal with emotions as they arise rather than storing them up.* Try to keep conflicts or disagreements current if you are to avoid major confrontations. Explosive situations arise because group members are unable or unwilling to handle emotional crises as they encounter them.

- *Challenge any attempts to rescue a member from a painful but perhaps necessary experience*: Some members consistently try to:

- Console/be kind
- Plaster over the cracks
- Sweep under the carpet
- Make everything better

If this is not explored, energy in the group can be dissipated and unhealthy behaviours can be institutionalized.

- *Do not allow gossip.* People in groups often talk about another (present) member as if he were not there. They talk to me or to someone else about the third person. I challenge this every time because it weakens and erodes many of the values and norms that we have been looking at. I encourage members to look at and address each other directly and use first names.

- *Avoid over-exposure.* Most people in groups will share and reveal themselves at their own pace. Sometimes, however, in the early stages of the group when people are unsure of the boundaries, an individual may reveal too much about himself or go too far. This can frighten other members who may feel they have to perform similarly. It can also be difficult for the individual who afterwards may feel embarrassed or regretful and can find it difficult to return to the group. To avoid this, work gradually and sensitively with people's feelings at the start. Check out constantly if it is alright for the person to continue. Are they making a choice to talk or feeling compelled to talk? How are other people feeling? Be aware of your own reactions to the person and trust your judgement.

- *Avoid 'why' questions.* Questions which start with 'why' are 'closed' in that they demand an explanation or a specific answer. They are rarely helpful and are best avoided. Questions which start with 'how' or 'what' are more valuable because they allow a person to be more 'open' about their experience or feelings. Use and encourage questions like:

- How is this for you?
- What is happening for you?
- How do you see/feel/experience things?
- What is it like for you?

These are present-tense questions. They open up the process and involve the person in their own experience.

Working with members' feelings in these ways will deepen and enhance the learning which takes place in the group. It will also be evident over time that members are developing healthier and more creative ways of relating to each other based on acknowledgement and acceptance of feeling and emotion. Feelings will come to be regarded as significant, desirable, and productive and will add to relationships instead of disrupting or detracting from them.

Teaching members how to maintain themselves

Every group is set up to achieve some tasks or goals which its members believe are worth striving for and yet it cannot devote all of its energy and resource to doing this. If the group is to achieve its goals and not fall apart on the way some of the collective resource must be invested in ensuring that members feel included and able to participate, are respected and valued. So from the start each group has to find a way of balancing and apportioning energy, resource, and time to its goal-oriented activity and to looking after its members.

Unfortunately few groups are able to create a healthy balance between their task and maintenance concerns. They frequently act as if these two needs are in opposition or competing for limited resources, instead of seeing them as essential and complementary. In this, most groups tend to reflect the larger societal preoccupation with striving, achievement, and success which is inculcated in the family and institutionalized in school and workplace. As a result many people will arrive in your group intent on getting on with the job and quite unskilled and uncreative in their ability to look after relationships. If this situation is allowed to develop the group can rapidly become a very unhealthy experience characterized by competition, apathy, or burn-out.

If you can identify some or all of the following behaviours and attitudes in your group and they do not seem to be obviously related to its stage of development then it is probable that your group is mishandling its task-maintenance needs and requires assistance:

- Tiredness, exhaustion, flatness, sense of being stuck
- Frustration, burn-out
- Conflict, bickering, arguing over goals, programme, resources
- Apathy, boredom, indifference, reluctance
- Absenteeism, lateness, drop-outs, turnover of members
- Poor concentration, decision making, problem solving, creativity
- Slow starts, never having enough time
- Excitability, tension, emotionality, irritability

Prevention is better than cure

I was once called in to work with a team of workers who were very exhausted and suffering from stress and burn-out. I found them to be very depressed and quite self-destructive and at a point where it was not possible to help them move on. After six months the team had to be broken up! I learned two important lessons in this group:

> • Help a group see the necessity of maintenance activity while it has a choice to take care of itself. When it reaches break-down it has no choice at all!
> • A group which can play together is more likely to be a group which can stay together!

Now when I work with a group I emphasize from the outset the importance of paying attention to maintaining and looking after relationships in the group if the job is to get done successfully. I introduce a more organic rhythm to the programme and to each session which balances and reconciles the task and maintenance needs in the group. This rhythm starts from the simple fact that every session has a beginning, a middle, and an end and draws attention to the needs of members at each of these phases.

Try to get into the way of viewing your sessions more organically. Do not simply pitch into work after an initial greeting or suddenly stop when you become aware that you have run over time. These are patterns of activity and relating that many people have picked up in school and the workplace and if allowed to develop unchecked in your group will create a very stressful and unhealthy atmosphere. Aim to start slowly giving people time to gather and settle down. Move gradually into the main work for the session and leave time to wind down and separate. Here are some things to consider.

Beginning: a stitch in time

A 'nurturing' beginning is best, so arrange seats if necessary (in a circle), check warmth of room, greet people as they come in, offer refreshments if this is appropriate. In every group I use the check-in procedure outlined on page 97. I ask people to say how they are feeling, what they have been doing since last session, what they are looking forward to in this session, and anything else which might be appropriate. This helps members:

- Include themselves
- Connect with each other
- Settle down
- Helps the leader assess the mood and feel of the group
- Gets everyone talking at the start
- Affirms each member as important and unique

If people come in late I will briefly review what has been happening or invite members to do so. It is usually worthwhile clearing up any unfinished or leftover business from the previous session which might get in the way, and going on to outline the activity for the day or provide a context for the session. If you find that:

- The check-in is shallow or empty
- The check-in goes on too long
- People are not really interested in each other
- People are waiting or stalling
- Some people want to get straight to work
- Some people are tired, flat, depressed

point this out to the group straight away and get them to consider possible consequences and coping strategies. Often I have found that I spend the rest of a session dealing with what was not discussed in the first five minutes.

Show people that they are important and that their anxieties and questions are worth group time. If people feel valued and accepted here they will carry these positive feelings into the next phase. Do not smother or patronize people or let this beginning stage drag on. Watch out for signs or comments that tell you people are ready and willing to move on.

The middle or formal work phase: a bad penny will always turn up

Ensure that members know what the activity and its purpose is. Check that tools, materials, resources are available if required, people understand their role and feel able to contribute. If you have adequately prepared the group for its work at this stage it is probable that difficulties which occur have got more to do with members' personal needs and relationships.

Watch out for:

- Members who are tired and need a break
- Members who are hungry or unwell
- People who may be overly enthusiastic or dominating and alienating others
- Members who are quiet or who may feel ignored, deprived, rejected
- Activity that is getting too complex, intellectual, or becoming bogged down in details, is becoming boring or unsatisfying
- The group working to unrealistic deadlines or with anxieties about time
- Only a few people contributing
- Asking too much of group members

Should any of these or other themes become apparent, the best thing to do is disregard the agenda for a while and draw attention to what is happening. Many group workers are very nervous about leaving the task to focus on the process or maintenance issues and prefer to ignore them, hoping it will all come right. This is usually a mistake. What is ignored will always come back to haunt the group so deal with issues as they arise.

Encourage members to acknowledge and respond to the needs behind a behaviour or incident which are being ignored or dismissed. Do not allow conversation to range widely or evoke fruitless resentments. Keep discussion focused on the particular incident and make sure that it is seen and dealt with as a group problem. Give yourself a time limit – fifteen minutes perhaps – to open up the important issues and make space for people to share their feelings and declare their interests. Do not look for instant resolution; very little can be immediately resolved in a group. It is more of a cumulative process. Be confident that you have acknowledged the difficulty, discussed it, and involved group members. This is usually enough to take the steam out of a situation and let you all get back to work.

The end of the session: don't pour gallons into pint pots . . .

It is surprising how many groups end suddenly, with little preparation for a return to the domestic environment and a sense of being cut off or left hanging in the air. This can have a counterproductive effect in the group and will often create fear, resentment, and stress. Make sure to leave some time at the end of the session:

- To wind down and relax
- To summarize, draw conclusions, complete, contextualize the session, tie up loose ends
- To plan the next session, unfinished business
- To appreciate and celebrate
- To prepare for re-entry into domestic environment

This seems fairly obvious and yet many workers forget to help the group wind down or simply run out of time. Another type of worker fails to see the importance of giving precious time to this and demands work right up until the bell.

The ending phase need not take up a lot of time and yet it can have far-reaching effects.

- It can minimize emotional fall-out from the session
- It can allow business to remain unfinished and held over to the next session
- It gives a psychologically necessary sense of achievement and completion
- It can prepare members to handle eventual group termination
- It teaches members to pace themselves and inculcates an organic and rhythmic aspect to group experience

The simplest method of ending is to invite each member in turn to check-out. This involves members reporting what they have remembered, learned, appreciated, or resented in the session. Often issues will come up at the last, or people will report feelings or experiences that could have been looked at earlier. It is important to acknowledge this but not to go into detail or allow yourself to be manipulated into running over the allotted time. Agree with people that this issue can go on the agenda for the next meeting. You might decide to go first or last and give your own summary of what was happening in the session. You can use other ways of ending the session – a game, exercise, piece of music, or some quiet contemplative time together.

By paying attention to the way in which members come together, settle down to work, and then end their session you will gradually inculcate in the group a feeling for a more balanced, compassionate, and graceful way of being together. Members' ability and willingness to work on their maintenance issues, and develop their team spirit and camaraderie all flow from your initial efforts to create a pattern and a context in which relationships are as important as the task.

Pleasure versus striving feelings

I said earlier that a group which plays together is more likely to stay together. What I am pointing to here is the importance of a group being able to celebrate its activity and achievement, do things, and take time out to enjoy and appreciate each other.

One way in which I help a group develop a sense of play and well-being is to introduce and help members distinguish between times when their pleasure or striving feelings are in the ascendant. Striving is about attachment to a goal and the need to achieve. It can bring pleasure but often it may become an end in itself and distorts and subjugates satisfaction so that a person may come to feel driven or compelled. Pleasure, on the other hand, is about the ways a person nourishes and nurtures himself and involves choice and self-affirmation.

Early in a group's life or when it seems appropriate, I will devote part of a session to exploring these two ideas. Members easily understand their essence and relevance and are quite able to identify their typical strategies around striving and gaining pleasure. I then help people look at how their striving patterns could lead to competition, dominance, and selfishness in the group and encourage them to think about the need to develop ways of managing anti-group behaviours as they arise. I also ensure to brainstorm or compile a list of things which would bring members pleasure, as from this the group can internalize the importance of maintenance and plan an appropriate programme of activity. Familiarity with the language and practice of pleasure and striving gives a valuable context within which to explore an issue, and means that afterwards members will naturally look for something that they can do which will be healing and affirming. It also legitimizes the creation and use of particular rituals or activities which give pleasure and satisfaction and provides a simple way of presenting the need to balance task and maintenance issues in the group.

As the group develops you will find that your early efforts to teach and instil the importance of maintenance bear fruit. Increasingly, members will be able to deal with disruptions or interference to the task, attend to relationships, and work together more creatively and harmoniously. The group will develop a tolerance for the pace and speeds of its different members and will come to relate and work together in a more organic and whole manner.

Teaching members how to analyse group process

Every group faces certain common problems – identifying goals, creating a comfortable climate, developing procedures, making decisions, and the like. It is valuable if members are able to recognize and discuss the processes which occur as they are happening because it makes for greater and more intelligent involvement and agreement. However, being able to recognize group process, quite apart from commenting on it, does not take place by itself and methods of analysis have to be built in, if members are to become able and willing to turn from *what* they are discussing to explore *how* it is being discussed. I use a number of methods to help members become more self-analytical.

Worker process comments

Initially the impetus for highlighting process or maintenance issues comes from you. By indicating your awareness and interest in what is going on you will:

- Illustrate how the sessions influence behaviour
- Indicate the immediate problems confronting the group
- Legitimize discussion of process
- Build in the process-analysis function as a feature of the group's activity

The important thing is to choose a suitable place to intervene and comment. Try to deal with the behaviour or activity of the group as a whole and avoid drawing attention to particular members. This makes it less threatening and easier to engage people. You are trying to encourage the group to examine what is happening, so make a short statement about what you see in front of you and then ask a question:

- 'We've spent longer on this decision than we agreed to. I wonder what's happening?'
- 'Everyone has been silent for so long now. How are people feeling right now?'
- 'No one is really saying anything new here. What's blocking us?'

At first members may ignore your comments or not speak because they are unsure how to respond or what to say. Permit this and help members look at their embarrassment or discomfort. As the group develops, your process comments will become more normal for members and will increasingly activate analysis of what is really happening in the sessions.

Member process comments

When I begin to remark on, and draw attention to group process, I introduce a basic ground rule:

Each member has the right and responsibility to comment on what is happening at any time in the group

---

As members begin to intervene at the process level you may notice that some comments are ignored, while others evoke anger or conflict. This can often arise because comments are too superficial or too threatening. In either case it can be valuable to spend time teaching the group how to give feedback (see page 133) and introduce some of the ideas about creating right relations (see page 168). The process interventions of members are not only important for their value in exploring what is happening in the group but for the opportunity they present to introduce ideas about, and practise the skills of communicating, working, and living together.

The process period

This is a period of time which is set aside or given over to assessing what has happened in the group or what is taking place in the present. In some groups I have found it useful to structure this into the session, for example, a training group, but in most groups I will suggest a process period in response to a difficulty or an incident. It is important to give a set time – between ten and forty minutes is best – so that members can see their explorations in the context of the session.

You can decide to encourage the whole group to work together or may opt for smaller sub-groups. The sub-groups encourage greater participation and can be given one aspect of the problem to consider and report back to the larger group. You can help the large group focus on process by using brainstorming techniques or exploring the critical incidents and sequence of events that led up to the conflict or impasse.

The process observer

Sometimes group members can get so caught up in their experience that it is difficult to help them step back and see the process at work. I find it valuable to use a 'process observer' at these very emotive times who can then 'officially' sit outside the events and report on what is occurring. It is important to thoroughly and specifically brief this member on his role and what he is to watch out for.

Ask the process observer to focus on the way the group makes decisions, communicates, or distributes power and consider giving a checklist, like the one overleaf, to assist him.

After a set time, say, ten or twenty minutes, the process observer can report back to the group what he has seen happening and this initiates a discussion about causes, strategies, and resolutions. It is important that the process observer is able to give feedback and not threaten particular members. This is usually a very popular activity and is worth considering as a way of introducing the idea of process analysis because of its value in engaging group members.

These simple methods if used singly or in combination can provide substantial insight for members about how they influence and

- Is everybody included/listened to/consulted?
- How does the group handle dissent/conflict?
- Are decisions consensual, majority vote, or individual?
- What was the group atmosphere like? (Note *when* it changes and *why*)
- Who makes suggestions, suggests procedures, compromises, rejects, asks for votes, disrupts, makes proposals, asks the others?
- How does each member hinder or help goal achievement?
- How far did the group get in achieving its goal?
- How could decision making/communication be improved?

are influenced by the group. They also encourage members to take responsibility for what happens between themselves and begin to identify the options, consequences, and choices for change. I believe this is one of the more exciting fruits of encouraging process analysis and members increasingly move from a passive to a pro-active stance in the group as they come to realize that they are in charge of their experience and perception.

Working with difficult situations

There are a number of difficult situations which crop up sooner or later in most groups and will require you to intervene at some stage.

Dominating member

The dominating member behaves in a way which will give him, or enable him to exercise, more power in the group.

Manifestations

- Constantly talking
- Having the 'worst' problems and therefore 'needing' attention
- Being the 'nicest' or 'kindest' person
- Knowing what is best – adviser, critic, 'leader', moralist
- Acting aggressively, attention-seeking

Some of the causes which contribute to one member taking over or dominating may include:

- Lack of trust
- Poor cohesion
- Feelings of inferiority or inadequacy
- Fear, anxiety, embarrassment about speaking out
- Unequal relationships, problems with distribution of power, knowledge, skill
- The dominator may feel superior, more able, needier, more distressed
- The dominator may feel afraid of silences

You may decide to wait until a crisis develops around the role of the dominant member or you can intervene at a suitable point before breakdown occurs. In either event:

- Acknowledge what is happening and make it a communal problem with consequences for the group. Do not allow one individual to be seen as the problem.
- Bring out whatever feelings are involved on all sides.
- Highlight the process by which the situation came about. Explore people's needs and motivations and look at what is missing, being avoided or made covert.
- Management structures may need to be introduced or over-hauled – speaking in turn, rotating leadership of sessions, timesharing, setting an agenda. It might be important to set up skill-training sessions to look at aspects of communication, trust, decision making, and the power structure in the group. Think about ways of reinforcing sharing behaviour and introduce values, norms which emphasize mutuality and reciprocity.

Getting stuck

Frequently one member or even the whole group can become stuck or locked in a particular feeling or behaviour.

Manifestations

> - Long or recurring silences
> - Resistance to advice or suggestion
> - Atmosphere which feels cold, frozen, flat, wooden, dead, tense, or unreal
> - Repetition of a particular feeling or behaviour
> - Taboo areas and subjects: sex, race, religion, politics, anger, competition, individualism
> - Difficulties in sharing, trusting, deciding, planning, working
> - Loss of creativity, productivity

Some of the causes of getting stuck include:

> - Unresolved feelings or issues
> - Member or group feeling in deep water, out of their depth, in unknown territory
> - Unexpressed feelings of anger, resentment, sadness, inadequacy
> - Collusive agreements to avoid dealing with problematic or painful material, issues, dynamics
> - Difficulty in trusting, joining in, sharing
> - Opposing or entrenched viewpoints, sub-groups, inequalities in relationships, power, knowledge, skill

As soon as you become aware that a member, or the group is stuck draw attention to what is happening. By now the procedure should be familiar – make being stuck a communal problem, bring out the different feelings involved, and through working on the process issues help people understand why they are stuck and what choices they have about it.

If members find it difficult to talk in the group consider dividing into pairs or threes for ten minutes to talk about the problem from a more individual perspective before coming back to report in the large group. Brainstorming singly, in pairs, or in the group is also valuable as is the 'sculpting' technique we looked at earlier (see page

143). This is a powerful way of exploring why a group is stuck and you can ask members to sculpt themselves in terms of themes like intimacy, power, competence, and the like. Do not forget to discuss this thoroughly afterwards. Anything which involves physical activity can be a very good way of breaking open a pattern of stuckness and releasing people to examine what is going on, and should be considered.

The cynic or sceptic

The cynical member sets himself apart from the other members by his disbelief and constant sneering at the possibilities in the group.

Manifestations

- Condescending or patronizing attitude towards worker/ members/group goals
- Scoffs or sneers at mutuality; professes to believe people are only motivated by self-interest
- Nit-picks, points out flaws, weaknesses of plans or inter-actions, constantly deflates and disparages
- Mocking, sarcastic, contemptuous behaviour

Some of the causes of cynical behaviour in the group result from:

- Bad or painful experiences in the past
- Fear of failure – the cynic doesn't try!
- Fear of intimacy and tenderness – cynicism is used as a defence against getting close

---

The cynic is quite touchy and easily alienated so I usually try to deal with him indirectly at first. When a member is cynical about a situation, interaction, or planned event, I invite him to explain his doubts to the other members. By making him responsible for his cynicism it is possible to eliminate much of the sarcasm and scoffing which goes with this attitude while at the same time creating a situation where a member's cynicism serves the group. Groups can get unrealistic and inflated about their intentions and exchanges so having a cynic around can ground people and draw attention to unconsidered deficiencies and shortcomings.

. If there is a chronic or very severe problem with cynicism in the group it should be confronted with particular reference to its separative and distancing functions. In extreme cases you may have to weigh the degree of cynicism against the group purpose and contract and ask a member to review or consider his involvement in the group. Generally, however, I find that if I maintain an open and friendly attitude to this member and convert his contributions, in time the cynic lets go of some defences against getting close and will allow himself to join in more of the group's activity.

What to do if someone breaks down

On very rare occasions you may find that a group member undergoes an emotional crisis or becomes very distressed. Here are some guidelines that you might find helpful in such a situation.

- The first thing to do is stay calm. Do not allow yourself to panic, blame yourself, or feel guilty. Most people experiencing distress are terrified of losing control and need to feel protected and contained. They will want to have confidence in you so decide that you are going to help and put everything else to one side.
- Listen to the person. Try to understand what is happening, what has triggered off this crisis. Do not rush in to make things better or rescue! Give yourself time and let the person tell you in their own way what is wrong. Do not try to deepen the experience by getting him to act out his feelings or try to do therapy with him. All you have to do is let him talk – you listen! When you know what is happening you can develop options and find a way out.
- Do not allow yourself to feel afraid of being useless or inadequate. No matter how distressed a person is there is always one part of him that is in touch with reality. Speak to that part and he will respond. If you find yourself getting stuck, get in touch with what you feel and think about it for a moment. Your feelings will probably mirror those of the distressed member and you can use them to get on his wavelength,

create boundary, ask questions, and generate options. Follow your hunches and feelings and do not be afraid to use your feelings of confusion or helplessness to open up the situation:

I'm confused about what you mean. Can you say that again?'

or

I'm not sure what is the best way to help you with this. Tell me why this is happening for you now.

Ask other members for their views and comments but do not let them analyse or make intellectual points about what is occurring.

- You may need to give the distressed member time after the session or get more expert help. Do not feel guilty if you have to refer the person on. You cannot be all things to all people.
- Help the other group members express their feelings about the situation at an appropriate time. They may be shocked or feel frightened and it is important to work through this if you are to avoid people dropping out or the group getting stuck. The distressed member may be embarrassed about returning to the group or members may be afraid to refer to the incident. It is important to talk about this. The more honest you are about what has occurred the less frightening it will be for all and the more quickly everyone can integrate and learn from the experience.

Review

- Creative groupwork is about making space for options and possibilities to emerge in the group.
- There are three basic skills involved:

    1   Knowing how to use yourself as a model.
    2   Knowing how to influence and co-operate with what is emerging.
    3   Being able to provide structure and foster desirable behaviour.

- You will need to learn how to work with feelings.

- Teach members how to maintain themselves.
- Involve members in exploring their own process.
- Give yourself time with difficult situations and make them communal problems.

Chapter 10

The techniques of creative groupwork

The experiential nature of group behaviour and learning requires the worker and members to engage in an interaction which, by its nature, touches on all aspects of the human experience. The quality and richness of this interaction is in part a product of the processes that the worker knowingly or unknowingly helps to initiate and the relevance of the methods or 'technology' used to assist the group achieve its ends and resolve its problems.

In the last few chapters I have talked about what I consider to be the essential processes and skills to introduce and co-operate with in your group. I now want to discuss some of the methods that make up a basic repertoire and form the 'tool-kit' that you use to work experientially in most group settings.

The tool-kit

I developed my own tool-kit empirically and out of my urgent need to help group members find a way around the frequent and inevitable ruptures in communication. These breakdowns usually seemed to occur because members had some problem conceptualizing an event or because there was a language barrier or an emotional difficulty that got in people's way. Often there was a great deal happening in the group, but somehow it did not seem to come out appropriately or it was hard to identify a coherent pattern. The constant struggle to come to terms with language and reason seemed to constrain and confuse situations and produce only exasperation and frustration. I began to raid any other field or discipline which offered me ideas or practical advice that could be modified to create a richer and more complete experience in my groups. Through trial and error I began to evolve methods and techniques which in time I found transposed to most group settings.

These methods include and are derived from:

- Role-play and simulation
- Art techniques
- Imaginative techniques
- Games and exercises
- Bodywork
- Expressive writing and journalling techniques

Gradually I developed a structure and terms of reference within which I and group members could tackle any situation that emerged. There are four basic principles underpinning this structure and they give context and rationale to the notion of a tool-kit which can be used with groups.

- Technique as metaphor
- Technique as experiential learning
- Technique as a way of involving the whole person in group experience
- Technique as a way of motivating people

Let us examine these four principles before we turn to explore the methods in detail.

Technique as metaphor

I once worked with a group of adolescent boys and girls who appeared to have mixed thoughts and feelings about each other which they were holding back and not expressing. Several attempts on my part to discuss the effect this behaviour was having on communication and trust levels in the group met with no success – members denied that there were hidden agendas in the group and would insist on moving on to other topics.

I decided to tackle this problem more indirectly and so in one session I invited the members to participate in an exercise designed to involve each of them. I divided the group and asked one half to role-play the members of a youth club committee whose responsibility was to administer the allocation and spending of a grant of £1,000. I gave each role-player a set of instructions which involved them in grossly caricatured alliances, collusions, and attempts to attract or dismiss each other but allowed them complete freedom as to how they did this. I asked the other half of the group to identify the secret motivations and agendas of the various role-players.

After an hilarious role-play we debriefed and discussed what had been occurring in the scene. Members talked about the obvious secrets of the role-players and explored some of the reasons why people might be fearful or unwilling to reveal their motives and agendas. Soon one member remarked that the role-play struck him as an exaggerated version of what took place in our own group. Other members agreed and quite quickly it was possible to bring into the open some of the feelings and sentiments which had previously been suppressed and begin to look at the factors involved in their suppression.

A number of points emerge from this example:

- Drawing attention to the facts does not always meet with members' agreement, elicit co-operation, or change attitudes.
- If you are dogmatic you can actually evoke in members a stubborn resistance or insistence on the false or unhealthy beliefs that you wish to change. This is why Paracelsus, that Renaissance magus, warns us against simply telling 'the naked truth'. The clever group worker should use 'images, allegories, figures, wondrous speech or other hidden, roundabout ways', to convey meaning and resolve difficult situations.[1]
- It is very possible to encourage people to explore their predicament by using a technique or exercise which is metaphorical, which simulates reality, and reveals the bones of a situation. Instruction by metaphor does not depend on an objective checking of the facts or on rational thinking. Instead, working metaphorically implies coming upon an actual situation from outside, intuitively and spontaneously, rather than from within the event through more usual processes of deliberation and logic, which can lead to protectionism and defence.
- Every method, exercise, or technique then as I use it, is a metaphor: a way of shifting perception and creating meaning. I am not interested in any medium or technique as an end in itself but

as a means of engaging people and providing a context for work, which is directly related to the members' level of ability and willingness to act. From this perspective the value of any technique lies not in its skill or knowledge base but in what it points to, its ability to act as a signpost, open up dialogue, and encapsulate meaning.

• This leads on to an important point – an exercise or technique which does not work is just as valuable as one which does. Let me explain. If I want to explore the need for trust in a group I can sit down and discuss the issue with members. Now this can become quite abstract since you cannot actually see or touch trust and in some groups this discussion may seem laboured. A much easier and more relevant method is to do an exercise with the group which, even if it breaks down, provides you with tangible material and rationale coming out of members' own direct experience and learning. In this way even a technique which does not work becomes an opportunity to explore the group process and develop new and agreed ways of working and behaving.

Technique as experiential learning

This last point is highlighting how you can use methods and exercises as a way of creating experiential learning in the group. Experiential learning simply means generating from personal experience, ideas, rules, and procedures which can guide behaviour and then modifying these concepts and practices to make them more effective, in the light of new experience. So in the example given above, the importance of being able to trust each other derives for members from their experience of what it is like to be together when there is suspicion or anxiety about personal safety in the group.

Experiential learning can be seen as involving four phases:

• Concrete personal experiences, are followed by
• observation, reaction, consideration, which leads to
• abstraction and conceptualizing of theory, principles, rules, and procedures, and
• application.

Experiential learning is based on three assumptions

- That group members learn best when they are personally involved in the learning experience
- That members must discover knowledge for themselves if it is to really mean anything to them
- That members will be committed to learning and working if they can set their own goals within a given framework

You can see how each method, exercise, or technique that you use in the group becomes an opportunity for members to experiment with new behaviour, try things out, develop, and practise new skills. Each exercise or technique carries with it the promise of learning when it is accompanied by consideration of the experience and analysis of its process. In this way your use of techniques and exercises becomes an organic and integral part of how group members learn and work and not some alien or gimmicky rite enacted at the start of a group or when you are at a loss as to what to do.

Technique as a way of involving the whole person

A basic premise throughout this work has been that every group is a multi-dimensional experience which must engage the individual at the physical, emotional, intuitive, and intellectual levels of his being. A moment's reflection reveals that not all individuals operate equally on all these levels in groups – some people may be comfortable or productive on one level rather than another. However, we do need access to all of these faculties and if learning and behaviour in the group is to be relevant and mature it is essential that you include and work with as many of these levels as possible.

Unfortunately many groups and workers often exhibit a style in which one mode of exercise comes to be overdeveloped at the expense of the others.

Thus:

- Some therapy groups consider the expression of feelings as the only valid form of work
- In some discussion groups verbal ability, conceptual skill, and high concentration spans are valued above anything else
- Some activity groups can become overly engrossed in the physical skills and dexterity required

The consequences of overdeveloping one level of experience in the group and neglecting the others can be far-reaching:

- Loss of creativity, depth, richness
- Getting stuck easily
- Boredom, repetition, superficiality
- Conflict, intolerance, tension
- Loss of productivity
- Reduced ability to learn
- Problems in expression and communication
- Development of elites and hierarchies based on skill, knowledge, or proficiency

If it is to be effective and creative each group must offer its members clear opportunities for direct personal participation and observation which will engage and evoke the whole person.

This means that the group leader:

- Must be comfortable and able to work with each of the major modes of experience
- Must be able to help members cross from one mode to another as appropriate
- Must be able to integrate the modes and involve the whole person

The more imaginative and expressive techniques – drama, art, fantasy are powerful and effective methods of evoking and utilizing maximum personal resource. They seem to build a bridge between the conscious self and unconscious elements and mediate between the rational mind and its more irrational, affective, and intuitive parts. They offer you very valuable methods of working through conflicts and balancing experience at the physical, emotional, and mental levels. In situations where it is often difficult for members to comprehend what is happening or verbalize about it, the judicious and discriminating use of these techniques can release energy, create awareness, and provide structure and context.

Technique as a way of motivating people

The truth of the matter is that you cannot motivate another person. Motivation is something that lies inside a person and not outside. It can be reached but not controlled. When you appear to motivate other people you are in fact tapping and aligning with motivations that already exist inside them. Motivation is about discovering and activating the highly personal desires of group members rather than producing them.

A motive is really a desire – a response to a felt need. It is desire that motivates and when you appear to motivate other people you are actually responding to their feelings in a way which enables them to gratify their desires while at the same time helping you to gratify some of yours. Real motivation is about the mutual satisfaction of desires.

You can use various techniques to boost the appeal of a subject or task and increase the motivational attraction for group members. Take, for example, work with a group of children where it might be important to talk about the principles involved in asserting oneself, saying no to a drink or cigarette or withstanding peer pressure to break into a shop. You are more likely to generate interest and enthusiasm for this project if it can be presented in a way which offers fun, activity, and opportunities for demonstration and exploration, as well as making the point. Members will be more involved and the experience will be more complete if you can create opportunities for them to tell a story, draw, or enact a role play which will bring out the essential principles.

So when considering a session or a theme in your programme have clear what you want to come out of it and then think for a moment about the range of desires that might be around for members. Refer back to Chapter 3 where Maslow's hierarchy of needs is discussed. When you have some idea of what people want, think about using an exercise or technique as a way of engaging members' interest and augmenting their reason for investing in the project. You might want to have another look at the subject of programming discussed in Chapter 2. The remainder of this chapter is given over to looking at some techniques that I have found very effective in group settings and that might be helpful to you. Also, refer to the extensive bibliography at the end of the book which lists useful books and anthologies of exercises.

Technique number 1

Using role-play in the group

Role-play is a technique that is increasingly used in the group setting to:

- Explore the role behaviour of an individual in a domestic, leisure, or work situation
- Practise new skills
- Explore and resolve a current problem
- Replay a childhood scene or fantasy situation

Role-play is a very flexible technique which can be adapted for work in any group setting[2]. In its simplest form, role-play involves setting up a scene which represents for an individual or the group, some conflict, anxiety, or need to practise new roles, behaviours, or skills. For example, a group member may be applying for a job and will want to rehearse the personal and social skills required to perform well at interview. Other group members will role-play people on the interviewing panel, boss, secretary, and the like and help the individual identify and become familiar with what he needs to do in this situation.

Here are some of the situations in which I have used role-play techniques in groups:

- An adolescent is anxious about an impending court appearance
- A child is confronted by a bully and does not know what to do
- An individual wishes to make friends with a particular male or female
- Resolving problems with parents/teachers/employers
- Helping individuals learn how to assert themselves/handle certain emotions
- Helping individuals learn and practise new social and professional roles/skills/behaviours
- Drawing attention to interpersonal behaviours and group processes – working with conflict, decision making, communication, trust, authority and control, sexuality
- Helping group members explore social, economic, and political problems

Why role-play is useful in a group

A working knowledge of role-play techniques is an invaluable aid to work in groups because:

- *Role-play increases involvement*: Role-play introduces and legitimizes a fun and alternative way of exploring difficulties or issues in the group. It encourages participation by group members and is an effective method of reducing tension and creating space to look at a problem. Often quiet or silent members will find it easier to join in and contribute to the work of a group when they can engage in a role-play which requires them to play a part rather than themselves. You can increase the likelihood of participation by allowing people time to prepare beforehand or giving them a script which they can refer to during the drama.
- *Role-play increases spontaneity*: Even in those situations where members prepare or start formally, the actors usually identify quite quickly with their parts and start to ad lib and improvise freely. This brings a creative and spontaneous dimension to the subject of the drama which frees people to respond to each

other in a more relevant and often intuitive way. There is often more immediate expression of feelings and a willingness to take risks which I find shifts interaction from a contrived or an intellectual level to one characterized by personal investment and authenticity. I have frequently heard members remark on the freshness, genuineness, and relevance of a particular role-play.

- *Role-play enhances awareness and understanding*: Frequently group members report an increase in understanding and empathy after they play the role of a significant other or observe a colleague play them in a scene. Exchanging roles increases a member's feeling for another person and encourages accept-ance of him. Often if there is interpersonal difficulty in the group I will encourage members to exchange roles in a repre-sentation of the incident. In the actual drama and in the review afterwards, members tend to be more accurate in their percep-tion and portrayal of what is happening, more sensitive to each other, and less anxious to prolong the conflict.
- *Role-play facilitates problem solving*: You can take any problem, relationship, or situation and create a role-play from the central elements involved. The flexibility of the technique means that you can stop scenes and discuss options, rework, alter scenes, try out different strategies and endings; all of which enhances creativity, risk taking, and problem solving.
- *Role-play deepens group cohesion and mutuality*: Because members can see everyone working together to solve individ-ual and collective problems, role-play is a valuable way of emphasizing and developing mutuality, interdependence, and goodwill. You can use it to nurture reciprocal helping rela-tionships and foster intimacy and acceptance of members' problems.

Guidelines for using role-play in the group

WHEN TO USE IT

Role-play may be used to explore any difficult or complex situation but it is most suitable when:

- A member is having trouble trying to describe a problem and the people involved
- A member is trying to clarify his relationship with a significant other
- There is an internal or interpersonal problem in the group
- Members need to practise or rehearse a skill or particular situation.

INTRODUCING THE ROLE-PLAY

Role-play can be presented as an impromptu opportunity to rehearse or try out new behaviours. In order to ground the role-play in people's experience, I relate it to a particular problem:

'Mary, it must be discouraging when your mother doesn't appear to believe that you can make your own decisions. If you like, we could help you practise talking to her. This might show you better ways of handling the situation and help you convince your mother that you are serious. Would you be interested in this?'

It is important not to make a fuss over role-play or to force members to participate. Present it as something which is interesting and useful and explain its potential in the situation.

HELP MEMBERS EXPRESS THEMSELVES

Help the member whose problem suggested role-playing, to describe the situation and the primary characters involved:

'First we must know who was involved in the situation and what they said and did so that you can select group members to play their roles.'

I encourage other members to ask questions and comment, in order to involve them and obtain the best possible picture of the situation. This also helps the initiating member increase his understanding of the event.

INVITE MEMBERS TO VOLUNTEER FOR ROLES

BRIEF ROLE-PLAYERS

I encourage role-players to make up whatever speech and action they believe best conveys how their character feels and behaves. When people are new to role-play I permit them to spend some time preparing their part or considering a script. However, once the drama starts members are instructed to express their character as best they can, using their own words and feelings, instead of sticking rigidly to a format.

Just before the scene starts, check that everyone understands their roles. Answer any questions and provide help where necessary. Agree a time limit for the action and then start.

DURING THE DRAMA

- You can stop the role-play at any stage to assess what is happening or what options are available.
- In some situations you may ask particular members to reverse roles in order to help someone express what he senses the other to be feeling. This is a very valuable little technique and can open up dialogue, create empathy, and awareness.
- Sometimes an actor feels unable to proceed or runs out of material. You can examine this in terms of what it says about the problem or you can enlist another actor or change to another scene. This sort of freedom helps people feel more secure and willing to join in.
- If you become aware that something is not being expressed between role-players it can be useful to ask other non-playing members to double for the particular people and say what they think is going on or not being expressed. I use this technique a lot and find it essential in opening up the fantasies and covert communication which role-play can draw attention to. It is also a lovely way of including every member of the group since you can put doubles on the role-players and even in some situations post doubles on the doubles.

AFTER THE DRAMA – DEBRIEF

The first thing you must do is de-role each player. Get them to say their proper name as this helps them step out of the part they have been playing. Frequently members can become very identified with their part and this may spill over into the session. I then go around each player and ask them to speak about:

> - How they felt, behaved in role
> - What they thought, felt about other roles
> - What they thought about their character
> - What they understand now about the situation

After this I invite non-playing members to comment. From the discussion that ensues, it is possible to highlight particular points, develop coping or skill strategies, and learn from the experience.

Do consider using role-play in your group. It need not take long – sometimes only a few minutes – and can be very valuable because of its potential for mobilizing group energy and resource.

Technique number 2

Using art and drawing in the group

Artwork is a term which I use to describe a series of collage, pictorial, graphic, or other media which enable group members to communicate symbolically. These techniques emphasize the feeling and intuitive aspects of personality and offer a valuable way of exploring events in the group life which are not always logical or are hard to talk about in a coherent way[3].

On occasion a group may not have the linguistic or conceptual ability to deal with an issue and if members are not to act inappropriately out of frustration or helplessness, it is important to provide them with a means of developing awareness about what is blocking them, strengthen their ability to cope with events, and facilitate the release of feelings. Various artistic and expressive techniques like painting, collage, and modelling lend themselves admirably to these objectives and it is important to be familiar with their use.

While at times I may use a wide range of media and artistic

techniques to help members express themselves, I find that drawing is usually the quickest and easiest medium to introduce and use in sessions. Drawing is a particularly good technique because

- Every aspect of group life can be portrayed and communicated visually even if it is only an angry slash on a page or the depiction of members as match-stick men
- Materials are basic and clean – pencils, crayons, felt-tips or ballpoint pens. Unlike paints they require no preparation or cleaning afterwards
- Drawing requires minimal skill or expertise and can penetrate to the heart of a situation immediately and spontaneously
- Drawing channels the emotional energy in a situation. It gives substance to what may otherwise be vague and uncomfortable and makes it possible to be more conscious and to talk about one's experience
- It builds a bridge between the verbal and the visual spheres, the rational and the intuitive mind, and the inner and outer worlds of experience
- Drawing is more evocative and revealing of members' experience than words. There is often less defensiveness and more depth in a drawing than in the words a person may use to describe an event

Here are some examples of how drawing can be used in group situations:

- To help people introduce themselves in a new group – self-portraits, self-advertisement, badge, motto, symbol for self
- To explore members' self perceptions – private and public self, masks, strengths and weaknesses, aspects of self, good and bad self
- To help members become familiar with emotions and feelings – quick line drawings of love, hate, anger, fear, etc., drawing opposites, brave/afraid, happy/unhappy, theme drawing on fear, etc., emotional masks, drawing feeling memories

- To explore family or interpersonal relationships – family portraits, sociograms, family trees, particular events or incidents
- To develop cohesion, co-operation, and working together – group drawings, team, and pairs drawing. Themes can include communication, group symbol or badge, sociograms, any aspect of life in the group
- To solve a problem, develop creativity or explore group process – drawing a particular theme, for example, how the group handles conflict, makes decisions, etc.; fantasy themes – life in outer space, draw a novel animal; make different drawings which represent a problematic situation, pictorial brainstorming, draw feelings generated by the incident

Guidelines for using drawing in the group

WHEN TO USE IT

Drawing can be used to facilitate or open up any aspect of group life or process but it is particularly useful when:

- A member is having trouble describing a problem
- Feelings and emotional material are getting in the way of expression
- Problem solving is blocked and members need access to intuition, imagination, and creative parts of themselves
- Members find it difficult to talk about or explore inter-personal relationships or group processes

INTRODUCING DRAWING

I usually introduce the practice of drawing early in the group's life when members are more open to new ideas. I follow a particular sequence which starts at the individual level and ends with members working together to produce something of relevance to the group. Initially I ask people to draw doodles, lines, squares, etc. and I counter assertions by members that they are not able to draw by asking them to use the hand they are most unfamiliar with. Abstract drawings in an awkward hand are usually enough to get everyone joining in since it now becomes permissible not to be artistic and makes it safe to put pen to paper.

From this I go on to asking people to draw more everyday objects and experiences, still in the unusual hand – telephone, flower, feelings, and the like. At a later stage I suggest that members pair up and I set them tasks which they must draw on a shared sheet – member A can draw circles and member B can draw squares, for example. These more abstract sketches involve people drawing in a non-threatening way and this helps them become used to working together. After a time it is quite easy to introduce themes such as 'time I stuck up for myself' or 'a situation which made me feel sad', which members can draw on the same sheet and talk about afterwards. I use a lot of these themes and tend to keep people in the same pairs in a session to deepen the experience and build intimacy, although over a number of sessions I rotate the pairings.

You can give more intimate and personal themes as members show themselves responsible and capable of working with them. From pairs I then move to sub-groups which can tackle various aspects of a theme such as communication. Each sub-group takes a topic such as non-verbal language, methods of communicating, or problems in communication and draws on a shared sheet whatever comes to mind on the subject. After ten minutes each sub-group presents its work verbally and visually to the others. When all the sub-groups are finished it is quite easy to have a group discussion about the particular theme because members have been stimulated, involved, and made more aware of their feelings and opinions.

The same process occurs in doing a group drawing on a theme. This time everyone joins in on a large shared sheet to visually brainstorm their thoughts and feelings about a subject. I start with innocent themes like shopping at the supermarkets or going to a party, before tackling more complex aspects of relationship or group process. By following a sequence like this over a few sessions it is easy to develop attitudes and approaches to drawing which are not based on needs to compete or be skilful but which see drawing as a valuable way of generating more information and involvement of members.

SHARING AND DISCUSSING THE DRAWINGS

It is very worthwhile to spend time after a drawing session in sharing and discussing. This is particularly important where you are using drawing to highlight process or open up a problem. Invite people to share their drawings – as much or as little as they wish. Do not insist on sharing! You can work in pairs or sub-groups initially, but do spend some time in the large group sharing and discussing. The questions in Chapters 8 and 9 will help you structure feedback and discussion. Avoid interpreting or imposing your beliefs about people's drawings and always try to evoke what the drawing means to its creator. You can usefully ask other people what it means for them, but the emphasis must be on their experience and associations to the picture rather than on its technical or artistic merits.

Think about using drawing in your group. You will find it an easy, valuable, and practical technique which transforms inner forces into visible shapes and creates conditions in which these visible shapes can then be transformed into ordinary words and understanding.

Technique number 3

Using imaginative techniques in the group

Imaginative techniques are ways of evoking and creating symbols and mental images to deal resourcefully with the problems and circumstances of group life. Often a group and its members may find the everyday mode of rational thinking more of an obstacle than an aid to understanding what is happening between them. In these situations it is fruitful to ask questions like:

- What colour is the group atmosphere right now?
- What image/picture/symbol comes to mind about what is happening now?
- If you were a fly on the wall how would you describe what is going on here?
- If you had a bird's eye view of this group/interaction/problem what would you see happening?
- If you were the ship's captain what would your first order to the crew be now?
- Imagine a wise person were available and willing to help you with this problem – what advice do you think he would give you?

On first sight these questions seem strange and you might imagine that it would be an awkward experience asking these of a group. And yet they are a powerful and natural means of evoking or drawing out feelings and experiences which already exist – though they may be hard to describe – and providing a structure and vehicle for their expression.

These questions employ the language of mental imagery and symbolism in order to help members connect to and communicate with areas of the self which can supplement and enhance the analytic mind. They consciously call up, or build an image to represent some aspect of individual or group experience and aim at focusing attention on the problem and increasing awareness and expression of personal experience.

Imaginative techniques include

- Visualization – seeing pictures, images in the mind's eye
- Guided fantasy – offering the individual or group a series of images which they can visualize and explore in imagination (see page 35)
- Symbolic imagery – images with deep symbolic meaning and regenerative properties such as the wise person, the path of life, water, sun, etc.
- Meditation – body relaxation, generating new ideas, insights, contemplative meditation

---

These techniques are based on two simple assumptions

- *Psychological energy and feeling can be channelled by a symbol or image, transformed by it, or integrated by it:* Roberto Assagioli, who developed psychosynthesis which uses imaginative techniques a great deal, believed that when someone was offered a symbol or situation to imagine, they projected thoughts, emotions and qualities onto it which came from their own experience.[4] This has obvious implications for work with groups, particularly in situations where members have difficulty expressing themselves or working out a problem.
- *Energy and behaviour follow thought:*[5] Visualizing a symbol, or any thought indeed, can lead to an identification with it and this can be used to establish new and more desirable attitudes

and behaviours in the group. When we create something we always create it first in a thought form. A thought always proceeds its manifestation. An artist first has an idea and then creates a picture. 'I think I'll make dinner' is the idea that precedes creating a meal. The idea is like a blueprint; it creates the image of the end product and then magnetizes or attracts physical energy to make the idea occur in reality, as the media advertising companies are very well aware.

So by visualizing or thinking about an idea or symbol, group members can create, vitalize, identify with, and evoke its potential and qualities in their interactions with each other. As you encourage them to observe the possibilities, the idea becomes more clearly defined. Feelings are attracted to it and the idea becomes a desire seeping into members' everyday experience. Thus by inculcating and developing thinking about teamwork, co-operation, sharing, goodwill, and the like you can help members gradually to create these very conditions in the group.

Here are some of the situations in which I have used imaginative techniques:

- Using symbols to explore group process – resistance, conflict, quality of communication/trust
- Using symbols to explore individual experience – body, personality, sexuality, relationships
- To help members identify changes which they would like to make in their lives, to make a decision or choice – useful exercises might be:
  1) Fantasy journey to the Temple of Silence[6]
  2) Encounter with the wise person/advice-giver[7]
  3) 'Ideal model', life/career/relationships, etc.[8]
- To evoke a desired situation and mentally rehearse skills and behaviours:
  a) Mixing socially with other people, making friends
  b) Asserting oneself
  c) Job interview, sports performance
  d) Training groups – professional performance and presentation of skills and behaviours

---

- To visualize and work through a difficult, frightening, or embarrassing situation in the future
  1) Making a speech, presentation, job interview
  2) Making friends, self-introduction
  3) Asserting oneself, ending a relationship, saying no
  4) Worst fears, phobias, and compulsions, shyness, stammering, blushing, drying up, getting stuck
- For healing and regeneration:
  a) Developing positive self-image
  b) Developing particular aspects of personality
  c) Relaxation and body awareness
  d) Overcoming illness or emotional disability
  e) Strengthening and developing the will
- To end a session and help members wind down and relax
- To develop creativity, problem solving, intuition, and imagination
- To promote norms and values in the group – sharing, mutuality, reciprocity, goodwill, etc.
- To help members evoke and connect to meaning, purpose, essence in their lives, work, relationships

Guidelines for using imaginative techniques in the group

WHEN TO USE

You can use imaginative techniques at any stage to explore individual or group experience but I find it best to use them:

- To help a member who is having difficulty describing a problem
- To channel feeling or emotional material which is obstructing expression
- To develop or augment problem-solving, creative imagination, intuition
- To teach members how to relax
- To help members mediate and confront reality
- To promote particular values, norms, and behaviours

INTRODUCING IMAGINATIVE TECHNIQUES

Familiarize your group with this way of working as early as you can and introduce the technique as an alternative way of understanding and thinking about situations. Ferrucci,[6] Whitmore,[9] Fugitt,[10] and De Mille[11] contain numerous exercises and imaginative activities that can be used in any group and will give you tips on how to introduce and modify this medium to your own particular setting. Do try to read these books if you can.

Some people like to participate in imaginative games with their eyes closed. Others prefer to keep their eyes open. Either is permissible but you may have to check that an eyes-open attitude does not indicate fear, suspicion, or distrust of the group or the medium[12]. Encourage people to be appropriately silent and not to talk or distract others. Initially a certain amount of talking and even giggling may be inevitable but if you persist with the approach, members will become accustomed to the need for silence and goodwill and respond accordingly.

AFTERWARDS

I often accompany imaginative work with drawing or writing. This serves to ground the experience and begin the process of manifestation and expression. Drawing or writing frequently unfolds other insights or ideas and is a valuable way of consolidating and making more complete the process of understanding. Sharing and discussion can then take place in twos, threes, or in the large group. You should try to relate the imaginative experiences to the here and now reality of the group. Ask members how and in what way the experience is reminiscent of or arises out of their everyday or group interaction. Do not force or insist on this because sometimes a person's imagery does not immediately speak to a situation and it may be that it only fits into place later. Usually, however, the experiences do contain simple answers and insights and will illuminate personal and group process with humour and grace.

Do consider using imaginative techniques in your group. You will find them not only a playful and creative way of working but a powerful medium for channelling psychological energy and generating new alternatives and solutions[13].

Technique number 4

Using games and exercises in the group

I was working in the first session of a group recently with professionals who wished to explore their practice with ex-psychiatric patients. People had introduced themselves but still the atmosphere was tense. I invited people to join me in some games and exercises as a way of breaking the ice. Group members proceeded to have a sword fight using their index fingers only, make statues out of each other, and have a conversation without words, amongst other games. This activity only took fifteen minutes and yet it was successful in reducing the tension and inhibition in the group and generating fun, excitement, and shared experience.

These and other games offer a valuable source of activities, exercises, and strategies for working with groups. They can be used and enjoyed by everyone as they usually involve simple and easily understood procedures. Here are some of the reasons for using games in groups:

- At the beginning of a group games can help people introduce themselves and become better acquainted
- Team games encourage members to do something successfully with others, promote trust, co-operation, teamwork, cohesion
- Communication games help members become aware of the importance of listening to each other, non-verbal language, and the various skills involved in self-expression
- Games can stimulate imagination, develop resourcefulness, and teach problem-solving and decision-making skills
- Games can help members develop awareness, sensitivity and control – when to be quiet, noisy, still, active, responsive to others, dependent, independent, interdependent
- Games teach the necessity of rules, procedure, and framework. They promote discipline, control, self-responsibility, teamwork, and the exercise of personal will and choice
- Games provide opportunity for fun, adventure, excitement, risk taking

- They generate interest and enthusiasm and can stimulate a group which is tired, bored, or just after lunch! Games help a boisterous or excited group channel and expend surplus energy
- Games involve physical contact, can enhance motor coordination, and develop poise, confidence, and self-esteem
- Games can simulate reality, aspects of group process, problems with relationships and can be used to explore dynamics and create resolution and meaning

You can see that while the objective may vary, I am interested in the purposeful and constructive use of games. Without a context or rationale, games are just a way of filling time or can be a frivolous, empty activity. I often come across workers who use games in their sessions but are vague as to why they do so. They may have attended a conference or course which started with the obligatory games session and believe this is how groups are supposed to be run. Other workers would like to use games as an alternative to more traditional verbal and conceptual ways of working but are uncertain as to how to do this.

Remember there are only four reasons why you should use games in a group:

- As a metaphor to simulate or represent reality.
- To generate experiential learning.
- To motivate people.
- To engage the whole person.

When your use of games arises out of one or more of these contexts then you will find that the game or exercise is relevant and meaningful and it is possible to use the game as a springboard to discussion, problem solving, or exploration of group process.

Guidelines for using games in the group

- *Build up a repertoire of games*: This will help you if the group is bored, tired, rowdy, shy. At the end of this book is a list of manuals and compilations of games which make profitable reading.[14] Over time you will develop a personal library of games which you can adapt to suit any particular occasion or need. Do remember to work out and rehearse a game before you try it in a session.

- *State the purpose of the game*: It is usually best to state the purpose and objective of the game in advance so that people have some idea of what they are getting into.
- *Invite participation*: Do not force or insist on members joining in. Members who sit out of a game are still involved through their laughter, enjoyment, encouragement, and appreciation of the others. Permit this and next time you will find them joining in.
- *Be positive and encouraging*: Maintain an attitude which asserts, 'you can do it, would you like to try?'
- *Time*: Allow adequate time for a game but pay close attention to how the group responds to it. A manual may advise twenty minutes but your group may only need half this time or may require more. So do not be afraid to improvise, change the rules, stop, or introduce another game. Remember boredom means trouble!
- *Review*: Most games benefit and enhance the work of the group if you devote some time afterwards to reviewing the experience with members (see page 226). Sometimes it is not appropriate or necessary to look at how members found the activity but as a general rule you should help members see the relevance and meaning of the games session to their work in the group.
- *Invite suggestions from members*: Many members will have experience of games or activities that they have found enjoyable and which can be easily adapted for the group. Not only does this more easily involve members but it provides you with material that you know works!
- *Always be sure you know why you are using a game or exercise*: If you cannot give members an explanation that makes sense then you should not be using a games approach. Make sure the game fits with what is happening and will lead to clarification.

A miscellany

Sculpting

Sculpting is a technique already referred to (Chapter 6, page 143). It can be used to explore themes such as intimacy, power, or relationships in the group. If used in a loose, flexible way it need not take up a lot of time and can be very effective in illuminating the interpersonal dynamics in a situation. Because it involves a spatial and emotional language rather than words or concepts it is a valuable tool to use at certain times in the group life.

I sometimes use sculpting with individuals in the group who may be experiencing some difficulty in describing a problem or incident. I will ask the person to assume a physical posture or gesture which expresses their feelings in the situation or conveys the main characteristics of the event. It can be valuable to include group members' comments on the posture as a way of helping the individual begin to articulate the experience. Sculpting can generate powerful emotions but with a willing and trusting group it is possible to deepen communication between members and heighten consciousness about the dynamics and processes involved.[15]

Creative writing

Some individuals and groups find writing a useful method of reflecting upon and expressing their experience. With these groups I often encourage people to write a few notes after an exercise or jot down their thoughts about an incident in the group as an aid to discussion. Encouraging members to keep a personal journal or establishing a group diary is another valuable method of helping people think about what is happening in the group and pick out the significant factors in a situation.

Creative writing is also a way of helping members communicate emotions which are often too painful or compacted to be released verbally and accustoming people to the expressive and cathartic value of image and metaphor. A technique that I find particularly effective in exploring a problem or some aspect of group process is to engage members in writing a group poem about the incident. The rules are simple – I write a first line pertaining to the situation and any member can then write any word, sentence, or lines which spontaneously come to mind. There is no attempt to create rhyme and the emphasis is on immediacy, intuition, and discovery. I have found this to be an excellent way of stimulating a quiet, silent, or withdrawn group.[16]

Storytelling

Many of the problematic features of a group can be dealt with through the medium of myth and storytelling. Sometimes an incident may be too painful or obscure to confront directly and inviting members to construct a story around the incident can be an effective way of expressing emotion and raising consciousness. You can ask willing members to supply one word in turn around the circle, a sentence, as much or as little as they wish to contribute. Storytelling can enhance conversation and communication skills and can be used to promote self-esteem, build confidence, and foster co-operation.

You can develop story making and narration by asking members to describe what they think is happening in photographs cut out of magazines, pictures on tarot cards, and the like. It is surprising how skilfully members can use the story method to uncover the elements of a situation and communicate with each other, when in other circumstances they might prefer to remain silent.

Music

At times I use music as a way of altering the mood of a group or channelling energy. An active group can be helped to relax by playing some suitably soft music and an inert group can find reggae or pop very energizing. Many group members have particular musical favourites and will respond to an invitation to share their musical memories with the others. This can augment exploration of a theme or problem and is an effective method of stimulating and generating discussion. The use of music also leads quite naturally to drama, role-play, and movement.

Developing a suitable climate for the use of techniques

When you first propose using role-play, drawing, visualization, or any game to explore group process, help members communicate and express themselves, you may encounter objections:

- I can't draw/act/do this
- This is stupid
- I don't like this
- What is the point of this?

It is important to allow these and other protestations and quietly point out that what you intend to introduce has nothing to do with the aesthetic or skill aspects of a particular medium. Clearly state your intentions and objectives so that people understand that they are participating in an experiential exercise which is for the purposes of learning, creating resolution, and meaning. Emphasize that:

- This is a different way of working in the group
- It is a way of developing more creative, imaginative responses to situations and problems
- There is no right or wrong, best or least. The emphasis is on inquiry, discovery, expression, and change

If objections persist you may have to give some time to exploring underlying issues in the group revolving around competition, exposure, trust, and confidentiality. Do allow for a certain amount of embarrassment or awkwardness as many group members may not be familiar with work involving modes other than the rational and verbal, and it will obviously take time and practice to become accustomed to some of these ideas.

You may find members acting in a provocative or undermining manner when they first try out these techniques. People may giggle, disrupt, or misbehave. Do not be put off by this! Most of us find new and unfamiliar situations threatening and behave similarly. Acknowledge the fear, embarrassment, or anxiety generated and repeat the technique in another session. Do not abandon the technique believing it is failing or is inappropriate. In most cases you will find that persistence creates familiarity and acceptance. Having said this, however, you must always respect members' freedom of choice about involvement in an activity. Participation should be on a voluntary basis and you should never force or coerce anyone into experiential work.

It can be valuable to agree a contract with group members determining the purpose of the exercise, the length of activity, how it is to be used, confidentiality, members' rights and responsibilities, and the like. This is usually sufficient to persuade even the more timid or suspicious members to join in. It is important to spend time reviewing and grounding the experience afterwards in order to evoke and articulate consciousness. Again no one should be forced to share and I usually preface this phase of experiential work by reminding members that they can share 'as much or as little' as they wish. The way in which you handle this review stage can determine how willing members will be to do this work again so be sensitive in eliciting feelings, question judiciously, and demonstrate that you are listening and appreciative of a member's experience.

You might wish to ask:

- Does anyone wish to share what that was like?
- How do you feel about what happened?
- What did you discover about yourself?
- Have you experienced anything like this before?
- What does this remind you of/suggest/what comes to mind?
- What does this experience say to you about what happens in the group/about your life?
- How can you use this experience to move on?
- What was missing?
- What could have been improved?
- What do we need as a group?

Through your questioning and your approach to the review of experiential work you can create an atmosphere which suggests that members are free to find their own way and that what they think and feel is fundamental. The review can become an opportunity to reflect and think critically, talk through issues, and try out new ideas, guesses, and hunches. This may be very exciting for members and can come to be positively associated with the new techniques.

Do not necessarily confine yourself to reviewing in the large group. Think about using pairs or sub-groups as an alternative to sharing and talking in the large group. The smaller units provide more time, opportunities for intimacy and depth, and a chance to practise conversation skills, empathy, and acceptance.

By being clear and open with members, firm, warm, and supportive, these techniques can come to be seen as an exciting and acceptable way of working mutually on group issues and personal concerns. Initial reluctance or embarrassment will come to be replaced by enthusiasm and satisfaction and your use of techniques will become an integral part of the way the group operates and a means of engaging the member in a creative and complete manner.

A postscript

It is clear that the variety of problems and situations encountered in working with groups is great and the actual methods adopted range widely. And yet the rationale remains the same – a vision of and belief in the power and creativity of fellowship, mutuality, and reciprocity. This leads me to believe that one technique alone underlies all efforts to work creatively with a group of individuals and help them achieve their personal and collective goals. This technique is based on love and understanding. The point can hardly be overstated.

Ultimately, vision is more important than techniques and methods. The group worker who has a thorough understanding of what happens whenever people come together and who knows how to co-operate with influence and allow these processes will be able to adjust his activities to the problems at hand rather than follow a prescribed technical procedure. Such a worker has a flexibility and creativity which has been acquired by building his work on principles and vision and not by memorizing routines and methods. Techniques are important, but they are meaningless and mechanized unless grounded in a vision of the possibilities inherent in fellowship and shared experience.

Review
- Techniques can be used metaphorically.
- Techniques are a way of generating experiential learning.
- Techniques are a way of motivating people.
- Techniques are a way of engaging the whole person.
- Techniques should be used purposefully and with intent.

- State an objective for the technique, invite participation, review the experience, contextualize the learning.
- Develop and build a repertoire of technique that can be adapted to any situation in the group.
- Remember that technique follows vision and goals!

Chapter 11

Working more intensively with groups: focus and context

In the last few chapters I have sketched out the essential processes and skills which I believe that you need to master in order to lead your group effectively. A knowledge of stages and patterns in group development has been outlined in Chapters 4–7 and process skills articulated in Chapter 9, which will enable you to be in tune with your group and intervene effectively, but I now want to draw attention to what underlies this. I want to turn now and consider the role and importance of the two practice skills which, as you become ever more familiar with them, will enable you to work more intensively and at deeper levels with your group and to include more of the members' preoccupations and concerns.

A central concern for the groupworker

It is clear by now that any group is a volatile, dynamic, and rapidly shifting system of individual and collective experiences and interactions, with multiple levels of need, activity, and performance. At times the group experience both for the members and the worker can seem and feel overwhelming, even incomprehensible, impulsive, random and, at worst, chaotic. Typically, at these times and in such situations a worker may be required to intervene in order to help group members clarify what is happening and make appropriate choices or assist in managing some change or event which is impacting on them.

A key problem for the groupworker is where and at what to direct his attention.

- What am I looking at?
- What does it mean?
- What is required of me/us now?

The question of what the worker pays attention to is about *focus*, and the question of making sense of the data or phenomenon observed is about how the worker creates a *context* for meaning. You may recall that I first mentioned the need for context in my introduction (page 2) when I said that context provides a frame of reference which informs and disciplines how and when you intervene. So, knowing what you are looking at and what it means provides the worker with the opportunity to intervene effectively and systematically throughout a spectrum of member preoccupations and concerns. We shall consider this spectrum of preoccupations shortly, but first I want to say some more about focus and context.

Focus is about:

• Attention	Noticing an effect, topic, feeling, behaviour, or its absence in the group or oneself.
• Observation	Studying for a time the *location* of the event; where is the centre of activity, the point of greatest energy? *Configuration*: what is the shape and size of activity? Who is involved and who is not? *Dynamics*: what are the feelings involved in the phenomenon? How does it develop or diminish?
• Definition	Is there a clear image, theme, or event which can be presented to the group for consideration?

Context is about:	
• Connection	Weaving together a mass of responses connecting events and behaviours which precede and follow a particular passage in the group.
• Reflection	Thinking about what is occurring both separately and collectively, creating words, sentences for what is happening, discussion, composition of themes and motifs, creating an hypothesis.
• Interpretation	Generating meaning, giving orientation, determining what the individual or group is preoccupied with.

Example of worker's use of focus and context in a group

A therapy group for adults had been meeting for about a year with a constant set of five members, when three new members joined.

They were well received by the old members, but after about six sessions I noticed that I was feeling vaguely dissatisfied with the quality of group interaction. I could not determine what my discontent was about so I set myself simply to observe for the next session or two what was occurring in the group.

What soon became clear was that there was really little interaction. Each member seemed to take a turn in presenting their current life experience to a seemingly attentive but silent audience. This was in marked contrast to the established pattern of more spontaneous and reciprocal interaction engaged in by the senior members before the new arrivals. It was clear that in some unspoken way the whole group – but in particular the large subgroup of senior members – were relating with each other in a manner which seemed to promise attention but not mutuality or engagement. I became more aware of a sense of impatience in myself with the senior members whom I thought should know better and should be inducting the newer members into the norms and ways of the group. I knew now that I had located a disturbance in the group and I had some sense of the size and shape and who was involved in that disturbance.

On thinking about my impatience with the lack of mutuality and my irritation with the senior members for withholding real contact while seeming to give attention, I began to conjecture that the senior members were punishing me for introducing new people while at the same time withholding the benefits of group experience from the invading arrivals, and that I was reacting to this. I now felt able to draw the group's attention to a clear theme of distant and uninvolved contact and invite discussion. The senior members in particular denied that they were uninvolved and asserted that they were only sharing out the group time so that everyone had a turn and that no one felt excluded. They were oblivious to the point that the emphasis on fair shares was not only about equity but must also indicate a fear of losing out to others and a defence against the wish to exclude the newcomers from getting more.

It was not possible to get much further with things until two sessions later, when two senior members missed the group session without notice and most untypically. Members who did attend worried that the absentees might not come back, though there were no grounds to believe this; they feared that the absentees were not getting enough from the group and became anxious that the group had got too big to provide everybody with what they needed.

When the two absentees turned up the following week with weak excuses for not attending, it was now much easier to invite reflection and discussion about what was really going on in the group as it was manifested in the quality of relationship and engagement.

Gradually, senior members began to reveal their displeasure with me for suddenly introducing three new members and not staggering the entrances over time. The experience of feeling swamped and no longer the focus of my attention had rekindled old feelings of anguish and rage at the thoughtlessness of parental figures, displacement by younger siblings, and the rivalries and family allegiances that this generated. This had been re-enacted in the group rather than spoken about and worked with.

With these revelations the group now had a context in which to speak about their feelings and experiences of change, loss of the familiar, new beginnings, disruptions, newcomers, and reorientation. Early experiences of change, loss and adaptation within the family were now seen to create a template which moulded individual response to similar experiences in later life. Only by talking about these experiences in the containing and permissive environment of the group which each member had to build and contribute to, could the individual be freed from repeating the old patterns and choose a novel response.

Investigative and facilitative attitude of the groupworker

You can see from this vignette that what enables the group members to move to a more mutual interaction is the persistence and capacity of the worker to ask the group to focus on a particular problem and put it in a context which generates some meaning and opens up possibilities for development. Focus and context are the two poles of an investigative attitude which characterizes what a group experience can offer an individual.

Focus draws attention to some phenomenon in the group life, and context provides a container for holding and generating sense and meaning for that phenomenon.

The groupworker is the representative of an investigative attitude which places singular importance on considering process issues. The worker is the embodiment of an ethic which is based on the idea that the essence of group membership is shared experience, and that anything which inhibits this development requires examination and discussion.

- The essence of the human being is social, not individual
- The essence of the group is shared experience
- The individual is part of a network of social processes (family, occupational, political, religious, etc.)
- Disturbance in these networks can be re-enacted in the current group
- The current group can help individuals become aware of their unhelpful patterns of social disturbance and make new choices

Over time, this function of inquiry and curiosity becomes distributed amongst the membership, as the worker emphasizes the active participation of all members and their involvement with each other.

There are a number of major concepts which contribute to the investigative attitude in the group (see page 233).

But here is the crucial one:

> • All events and incidents in the group can be viewed as types and forms of communication, both conscious and unconscious, verbal and behavioural. These communications can be focused upon by the worker and members, and contextualized in order to make meaningful and exchangeable interaction.

We can even identify different contexts and levels of communication which can help provide the worker with an initial frame of reference and guide.

These contexts for group behaviour are characterized by decreasing awareness and ability to think and talk about what is really preoccupying members and an increased propensity to act out the core issues behaviourally:

The explicit context

The group is a public forum where everyone can see and be seen by everyone else. To enter a group, an individual surrenders some degree of privacy and autonomy, and that brings with it a fear of rejection and a wish to conform to hypothesized or explicit norms and values and real or imagined authority. So one often sees in the group individual members asking for permission to speak or apologizing for themselves – 'Can I just say . . .?'; 'I don't mean to upset the apple cart but . . .'. These and other protective and controlling measures were first learned in the family and school as part of the process of social conditioning and soon become evident in ordinary group interaction.

It is possible for the worker to recognize and categorize these explicit and conscious communications of members as operating within a context which is to do with and influenced by members' concerns about public opinion, social standing, and self-esteem, community, authority, law, custom, and the like.

The transference context

Transference is a psychoanalytic concept which refers to the tendency of individuals in an unusual or clinical setting to relate and treat others as if they were significant figures from their personal history.[1] So group members might relate to the worker as if to a parental figure rather than as a person in their own right or to each other as if they were siblings rather than colleagues.

Since the first group is the family group, all groups thereafter resonate to some degree with the dynamics, tensions, and yearnings of the primary group experience. The individual has to manage the presence of others in the current group as the inevitable struggles for dominance and status can so easily ignite re-enactments of the sibling rivalries of the primary family group. Members will compete with each other for the worker's attention, become preoccupied with the identity of the 'favourites' in the group, and show surprising sensitivity and jealousy around the worker's interactions in ways which re-enact and are reminiscent of earlier child–parent–sibling relationships.

When such behaviours and communications surface in the group, it is invaluable for the worker to have an understanding of the inevitability and almost 'normal' nature of transference phenomena in order to provide that containing and reassuring context which relieves the pressure and encourages members to think and talk about what is happening.

The projection context

'Projection' is another psychoanalytic term which refers to an individual's unconscious tendency to disown unacceptable parts of themselves for fear of being rejected.[2] These unwanted qualities – like anger or desire – or unacceptable parts of the self – like the clingy child or flirt or bully – are then projected onto others, who are often reproached for the very things feared in oneself.

I think that much of the difficult and intensive work in groups is really about working with these projections – so pervasive, mobile, and slippery. The desire in the group is to present a good image, and since group involvement entails a loss of privacy, individuals engage in a great deal of projection in order to hide shameful or unacceptable parts of themselves. Much of the worker's intervention in these circumstances is aimed at demonstrating to individuals and the group how they create situations where expectations and predictions about the world are fulfilled.

Once the self-fulfilling prophecies can be illustrated, work can then begin to help members accept the repressed primitive and instinctual parts of themselves and abandon the self-hatred and fear which gives rise to projection in the first place.

What helps me identify the presence of projective activity is to think of the group as a hall of mirrors in which everybody sees themselves reflected by the others present. Members can see others reacting to events in the same manner in which they do, or in marked contrast to their own behaviour. Often members will comment on this: 'You remind me of how I used to be . . .'. Frequently you will hear people say, 'You know it's like looking in a mirror . . .'. Sometimes these mirror reflections are helpful and enable members to get to know themselves through seeing the effect they have on others and the pictures they form of themselves. Sometimes the mirror reflections are so distorted or alien that empathy and contact are impossible and confusion and conflict are the prevailing moods in the group.

The worker endeavours to help members realize that it is parts of the self and not the whole of oneself that are being reflected, and that the power of the group is its capacity to provide different angles, perspectives, and levels so that one cannot avoid seeing oneself through others' eyes.

It is the unique property of the group that quite quickly it can provide each individual with a multiplicity of self-reflection – a picture in the round, so to speak – a refracted picture of oneself to reflect upon and consider, in any one moment immeasurably more complex and multi-layered than the simple view of one's own self up to that point. Through proximity and contact with others, the possibility emerges of correcting distorted images of oneself and discovering new dimensions and depths in one's being. But this is always a painful process and groups need a lot of training in order to understand and contextualize their behaviour at this level. The worker must always be alert and vigilant for how members are using each other and the group to deal with inner parts of themselves.

The somatic context

At times you may hear members talking about their experience of the group in somatic or bodily terms. Frequently, members will report how some emotional conflict or event in the last session made them feel sick afterwards. Another member will angrily describe how all this talking is giving her a sore head or the lack of co-operation is a real pain. Often, in a new beginning group, members will report sweaty palms, butterflies in the tummy, heart palpitations, and other physical sensations prior to talking or speaking out. It is as if the member's experience of group life is operating at a very primal and direct level and is expressed in physical terms.

People may perceive or experience group involvement as doing something to them somatically and producing painful or uncomfortable symptoms or making them worse in some physical way.

What is happening is simply that a very common experience for us all in times of crisis or emergency is being magnified in the group setting. In a highly charged or stressful situation people regress to primitive functioning in order to cope with or manage the real or perceived threat. We are all familiar with the instinctual nature of the fight–flight phenomenon. Now, in a group situation there is a loss of privacy, the experience of being in the public gaze, and the ever-present sensation of feelings swirling around and being amplified and magnified.

If something is happening in the group which is new for us or threatens our vulnerabilities, like introducing oneself to strangers or finding oneself part of a quarrel, we can respond to the heightened emotionality of the encounter with feelings of panic. It is these feelings of panic that engender the instinctual and reflexive nature of fight–flight responses, because panic undermines and attacks our capacity to think about what is happening. Not being able to think coherently about what is going on results in members feeling flooded with feelings and sensations, leading to that hypersensitive awareness in which the group is misguidedly believed to be causing the individuals pain and distress.

I will say more about this somatic context of group life and behaviour later (page 259) but for now I just want to suggest that you need to learn to recognize that individuals and groups do operate at these sorts of levels and that it is an entirely natural feature of group life which must be allowed for by the worker. I said in my introduction (page 4) that the group is organic and natural and that the group is an energetic experience. This means that there is ebb and flow in the condition and quality of the process and that the group can be emotionally and physically experienced and lived. This is why often, in interviewing individuals for prospective membership, you will come across fears of contamination and contagion and fantasies about the group swamping the individual.

Just as these fears and fantasies are dealt with in individual sessions by bringing them out into the open where they can be discussed and tested, so in the group the worker has to normalize these somatic phenomena and, by going towards them with interest and attention, recontextualize the circumstances as something to be explored and talked about rather than being overwhelmed by.

The archetypal context

The concept of the Collective Unconscious was developed by Carl Jung and represents a landmark in the history of psychology.[3] Before Jung, psychoanalysis had concerned itself exclusively with the exploration of the personal and individual unconscious.

Jung then showed the great extent of collective psychic elements and forces which exercise a powerful effect on the human personality. According to Jung, the collective unconscious is a vast world stretching from the biological to the spiritual level, and contains latent memory traces of human ancestral development. This psychological residue of evolutionary development manifests in patterns or predispositions which can determine the individual's response to life experiences and even what sort of experiences he has.

These predispositions or blueprints are called 'archetypes', and are the crystallization of human experience over countless generations. They appear in the human psyche as a readiness to behave and experience life along broad lines, themes or motifs.

The importance for the groupworker of the collective unconscious and its archetypal energies is that the individual is now linked not just to the past of his infancy but to the past of his tribe, culture, and species. This means that both the individual and the group are resonating to cultural and tribal symbols, stories, and myths, and that these impact on group life, shape it, and can serve it if the worker is tuned in to this particular context.

One of the first archetypal manifestations of the collective unconscious in any group is the scapegoat and its close cousin the sacrificial lamb. You may know that the scapegoat as a phenomenon dates from biblical times, when the wandering Jewish tribes used the animal actually to bear the burden of the sins of the tribe.

The scapegoat was then separated and exiled from the tribal group and sent into the desert to die. By contrast, the sacrificial lamb was not banished from the group but offered up on behalf of the group to appease God. The sacrificial lamb was therefore a martyr within and for the group.

What this all means is that groups throughout history and up to the present day share certain recurring dilemmas and tend to come up with identical solutions.

Indeed, I would assert that group involvement and membership centres on a core dilemma which can be stated thus:

> Being a member of a group requires an individual to surrender part of their autonomy in service of the whole but not to surrender so much that they merge with or are overwhelmed by the group, whilst at the same time asserting their individuality but not in such a way that they are alienated from the group or narcissistically preoccupied with themselves at the expense of group involvement.

The tensions for individuals and groups which ensue from trying to solve this dilemma are such that, inevitably, conflicts around dependency, independence, desire, status, power, sex, property, and the myriad of human concerns have to be spilt into good and bad parts and acceptable and unacceptable qualities.

As we saw earlier, the easiest way of coping with perceived negative or shameful impulses and desires is to project them into others selected for that purpose. People look for others to blame so as to avoid the pain of responsibility or the helplessness of need. So the scapegoat is invoked in the member who embodies the negative or disowned aspects of group life.

The scapegoat is always somehow different and in some way – because of age, gender, colour, religion, or point of personality – goes against the implicit or explicit rules of the group and is easily selected to bear the 'sins' of the group. By attacking and exiling the scapegoat the group membership hopes to absolve itself from its own unacknowledged and often secretly longed-for desires.

In the case of the sacrificial lamb, a member offers himself as a martyr for the group. Such a member may carry the group's aggressive feelings about the leader and engage in a hostile relationship with the worker until the behaviour is understood and contextualized. All sorts of resistances and ambivalent feelings in the group can be taken up and suffered by the sacrificial lamb, resulting in much misunderstanding and lost opportunities until such time as the worker can see what is really happening.

There are all sorts of archetypal patterns and motifs which are evoked and which influence groups. For example, most people as they settle into the group have a sense of journeying towards some goal, and a means I have consistently found helpful in contextualizing and illuminating the dynamics of a group in question is, at an appropriate stage, to invite the group to examine the story of the Wizard of Oz and find correspondences with this story and their own experiences.

You may recall that the story is about isolated individuals who, feeling a lack of something essential in themselves, band together to seek out a wise person who will help them regain that which they have lost. In the coming together, the individuals learn to care for each other, protect each other, and look out for each other – the very qualities that were perceived to have been lost! The wizard turns out not to be an expert but a man of compassion and good intent who tries to help the companions as best he can. Through his efforts the travellers learn to work and live together as a group, which in effect requires them to recover their lost qualities in service of the whole. This is a wonderful metaphor for groundwork, and provides a joyful context in which members can situate their woundedness and isolation and both identify with the various characters and be inspired to continue with the journey and its perils and hazards.

This is the power of the archetypal context for working with certain dynamics in groups. The archetypal dimension can be utilized to contextualize and transform behaviours and feelings which otherwise would bring chaos to the group. The aggressive member can be seen in the context of the warrior, and taught to respect their capacity for aggression and use it in service of what is valuable rather then waste it in petty squabbling. The attention-seeking member may be misusing the hero archetype. The member who monopolizes and dominates the dialogue may need some help to connect to the poet/bard or storyteller archetype.

The archetypal motif of birth–death–rebirth gives context and meaning to the experience of beginnings and endings, and members leaving and joining the group. I like to incorporate the old Pagan and Christian festivals of Halloween, Christmas, and Easter as part of the sense of rhythm and development in the group year.

The important thing to be aware of when including the archetypal perspective in your work is the interactional synchrony between the collective unconscious and the individual. Individuals in the group are acting out their own personal needs as well as replicating and re-enacting great mytho-poetic dramas and stories. And at the same time, collective myths serve the evolutionary process of the group and are re-embodied through individual action.

Use of the worker's self to provide focus and context

At the beginning of a group few members have much understanding of the power and value and the opportunities offered by the group experience, nor can they be expected to have much sense of community. So they need quite a bit of help in order to come together and intermesh. Initially, the worker accepts leadership responsibility as a way of:

- Engaging, motivating, and encouraging new members
- Defining the purpose of the group
- Clarifying expectations about what is possible, what is not, what is required, what is not

---

in order to:

- Create commonality, collaboration, and community

Because the essential property of the group is shared experience, the worker endeavours gradually to wean the members from their early dependency on him. The power of the leader is based on projections onto him of parental and authority images and experiences in each member's personality, and their expectations that the worker will behave in the traditional hierarchical mode of authority and leadership. Rather than fight this the worker accepts it as natural and appropriate, but slowly, and at the group's pace, moves in the direction of leadership which is more collaborative and participative. In this way leadership becomes more a function of membership than the automatic preserve of one person. The group learns to replace the worker's authority with that of the group and its members, thereby subtly modifying attitudes to and the exercise of authority.

The worker modifies traditional attitudes to authority among members and helps to deepen and intensify the group experience by:

- Modelling new positions
- Sensitizing members psychologically
- Acting as a catalyst to activate and mobilize what is latent in the group

The worker aims to foster the development of a shared psychic life in which everyone participates, to which everyone contributes, and for which everyone is responsible.

This means cultivating and emphasizing the investigative attitude which I referred to earlier (page 233):

- Group relationships could not exist or be made visible without communication
- Anything at all in a group which can be observed, perceived, or reacted to is a communication
- The groupworker is open to all and any communication which will locate and clarify what is really going on in the group

But especially:

- Relationships formed with the worker and other members are also the object of communication and investigation

This is to focus on the worker and member relationships and to use them as a context for inquiry and understanding and working with deeper issues of group process. This is a very radical and catalytic position which the worker adopts, and one which at times proves irritating and uncomfortable for most, if not all groups. Most people enter a group of whatever kind with some conflicts and problems around managing relationships. Participation in a group over time generates the desire for intimacy with others, but as these feelings arise members can become anxious about them.

You may recall that I said on page 239 that a core dilemma in groups was how to get close but not too close, and how to be separate but not too separate.

To resolve this dilemma, members throw up their characteristic defences against the disturbing feelings and as part of the process they may stop people getting close to them. However, the commitment to the group contract requires them to attend and not to flee the threatening relationships, as previously outside the group they might have done. What now happens is that the group becomes permeated with members' typical devices for avoiding intimacy and sabotaging relationships, because whatever defences are employed outside the group become manifest and re-enacted in the group. This material is what the worker repeatedly draws attention to and what members find so difficult to engage with, because if the group is to achieve its goal, members need to assume responsibility for the difficulties and complexities of group interaction and take some time to engage with and investigate the group process.

The worker's emphasis and insistence on deeper and more intensive examination of the problems thrown up by belonging to a group can activate rebellion and exaggerated independence in some members, compliance and dependence in others and this can stimulate the emergence of transference relationships to the leader.

Part of the worker's function is to be a transference figure, and it is the worker's understanding of his role as a transference object and his willingness to take on and focus on the transferences as a context, in order that they can be worked through and dissolved, that contributes so much to the group's capacity to transform member attitudes towards power, authority, and self-responsibility.

We will take up this theme of the transference relationships again in terms of how to work with them in the next chapter, but I want to now consider how the necessary self-examination of the worker in the group is another vital source of focus and context.

Here is an important principle:

- What characterizes and distinguishes the groupworker is his capacity to be both in the process and able to reflect upon it

---

The groupworker is not outside the group looking in, but is a part of the group – a member with particular administrative and process responsibilities. I have continually emphasized the capacity for shared experience as the central property of the group, and such an idea is based on the belief that worker and members alike are inextricably linked with one another in a psychic system which they co-create.

This is what is meant by the very useful concept of Matrix, which is a term derived from the discipline of group analysis and refers to the existence of a web of intra-psychic and interpersonal inter-relationships which grow in the group over time and which every-one in the group shares in, contributes to, and is influenced by.[4]

The group matrix consists of interacting processes between a number of closely linked and interlocking people and inevitably gives rise to the phenomenon of Resonance, which simply means that all group members, including the worker, intuitively and unconsciously tune into each other and to the relevant preoccupations and concerns of the group.[5]

This means that, since the worker influences and shapes the matrix and the pattern that the group takes and is also impacted on by the presence of the others, the feelings, hunches, intuitions and fantasies of the worker can, on reflection, provide important clues about:

- The internal life of the group
- What is not being spoken about
- What is not being thought about
- What is fearsome and to be avoided
- How members are feeling
- Why they might be feeling this
- What the anger/silence/depression might be about
- What members might be thinking about
- Why the group is stuck
- Why a behaviour/event is being repeated
- What the loss of creativity means
- Why there is difficulty sharing/trusting/deciding/working together
- What is happening between people
- What is not happening between people
- What is unfinished
- What is trying to emerge in the group

The mental, emotional and instinctual responses of the worker in the group are profoundly important and not to be ignored or discarded. I would encourage you to cultivate your inner awareness of your impressions and reactions, and try to think about them as a way of focusing on the group. This requires time, patience, and great effort and discipline to build and maintain skills of self-examination and scrutiny so that they become second nature. This skill of self-analysis in the context of the group is akin to the use of the counter-transference as a therapeutic tool by the psychotherapist or psychoanalyst.[6]

Counter-transference originally referred to the feelings and conflicts stirred up in the therapist as a result of working with the client and was seen as a obstacle to be eliminated.

Just as transference was held to be unfinished business from the client's family history which got in the way of things and required dissolving, so counter-transference was seen to be the therapist's infantile reaction to the client, which equally needed to be dissolved. In recent years, counter-transference has come to have a broader meaning, which includes the therapist's conscious and appropriate emotional reactions to the client and has been recognized as an extremely valuable clue about how the client typically reacts with others and the sorts of responses which he generates in others.

Like any powerful tool, counter-transference is a difficult instrument to master and effectively depends on the worker's ability to be empathic and to be aware of and in contact with his emotions without defending too vigorously against whatever unpleasantness might arise.

Example I

A woman in one of my therapy groups reported that she had recently attended a weekend personal growth group even though she knew that this was contrary to the rules of the therapy group which did not permit such extra-curricular activities. I found myself annoyed with her for this breach, and irritated with the other members who knew of the rule and did not challenge her on this. This happened on a second and a third occasion, and I found myself angry with the rebellious woman and the passive and acquiescent members. I refrained from saying anything because I wanted the members to confront her and because I did not want to appear the omnipresent authority.

When the third occasion occurred without challenge from the group I felt very angry with everyone and felt I had to say something. I did not know what to say except to be angry but I felt if I expressed my anger I would be going along with something unclear. At this point I tried to think about things and ask myself some questions:

- What on earth is happening here?
- Why am I so angry?
- Because the woman is breaking the group rule and provoking me
- Because the other members are going along with it
- Why is she provoking me?
- I don't know, but I feel like a father telling his adolescent daughter to be home by midnight and she keeps pushing the boundary

At this point I experienced immense relief because I had a possible context in which I could locate my anger and make some sense of what the woman and the group were doing. I told the woman that I was angry with her for the boundary breach but that I was curious as to why, knowing the rule, she would want to provoke me, and said that I felt like a father trying to curb his daughter. She replied that she too had been thinking why she had broken the rule and that I must be reading her mind because she had found herself thinking about her adolescent struggles with her father. We were now able to discuss her behaviour in this context and examine how she still reacted to authority figures today in the same inappropriate ways.

What also became apparent as the others took up this theme was how the group members were acting like younger siblings and letting this elder sister question and push the family rules and boundaries.

Example 2

This is the third session of a support group for staff in a young persons' residential home, and two female members of staff are talking about the strain of caring for their own children at home and looking after the disturbed adolescents in the unit.

They describe their guilt and the stress at leaving their own children at home and their sense of failing the young people in the unit.

The worker's internal response was as follows: 'I feel depressed and quite overwhelmed and find myself thinking about these staff as burdened and drained mothers who cannot get it right with their children.'

Two of the male staff join in and talk about how badly treated they feel by the young people in the unit and how they want to master the violent behaviour of the kids. One man produces the image of Ranulph Fiennes, the Arctic explorer, trekking across the icy wastes, pulling his own food, losing 5 stone in body weight, suffering severe frostbite. There are references to the mother of one youngster being 'a cold fish', and someone speaks of the suicide of a young man 'numbing' his key worker.

The worker's internal response was this: 'I find myself cold and aware of the absence of warmth, love and contact that these workers must encounter with certain young people. That leads me to think about the masochistic doggedness and determination that the explorer of the frozen human soul must endure in order to make contact. The other side of this is perhaps how these workers must deep-freeze their rage at their charges and even turn the fury against themselves. I feel quite helpless and think that I have nothing to offer this team.'

The deputy team leader comes in to say that there are consequences to bad behaviour and that the team should be united in their determination not to accept violence. This brings a painful and angry response from the key worker of the young suicide that, if the team cannot accept and deal with violence, then it is not surprising that the youngsters will turn it on themselves.

The worker decides to intervene at this point to share his feelings of impotence and helplessness at listening to the team's agony, and wonders aloud if such feelings of desperation are perhaps normal and natural in the presence of such human misery as they have to deal with. The worker suggests that if the wish to help another is rebuffed, then the desire to care can become an intolerable burden and, when combined with the struggle not to retaliate, can leave one drained and wanting to keep one's distance.

This intervention seems to strike a chord with members and leads to a discussion centring on the profound difficulties involved in loving and supporting youngsters who behave terribly and appear to kill off the very warmth and contact that they crave. The discussion is marked by a new quality of compassion for themselves in this work and for their charges.

Now, the point of these examples is to show how the worker cannot avoid resonating to the emotional undercurrents in the group and how, rather than ignoring these responses, one can actually use them:

- To reach a deeper empathy with the group
- To identify themes and preoccupations
- To pick out the prevailing feelings
- To develop possible interventions
- To create a context which the group can use

You may see different interventions from those that I made. What is important is how the worker allows the group matrix to enter him in order to empathize and understand. By working in this way the group leader receives the messages and communications of the group but does not get helplessly caught up in them and embodies and models the opportunity offered by groupwork to work together in a way which can transform individual and collective experience.

Here are some questions to ask yourself at difficult points in the group:

- What is happening to me at the moment?
- What do I see going on in the group?
- Why can't I think right now?
- What are people feeling?
- What am I feeling?
- What happened in the group just before this?
- What is trying to emerge right now?
- What does this member/the group need now?
- What do I need now?
- What is missing/being avoided?
- How is the group using me?
- Who am I now for the group?
- What does this remind me of?
- What is the myth/story/film script/song operating here?
- Who is silent? Can they offer anything?

This may seem like a lot of work and some people may feel that it is deserting the group *in extremis*, but there are times when it is vital that the worker step back in order to think about what is happening. The worker is the guide for members and you are modelling very important psychological and social skills. The group will continue whilst you are deliberating, and your silence and musing will gradually become familiar and the group will internalize this capacity for themselves over time.

By inhibiting your impulse to intervene hurriedly, you can create a space in which to think about some very unthinkable and unspeakable things and prevent yourself responding to an event in a way which justifies the member or group behaving in this manner.

Here are some typical counter-transference reactions that I find repeatedly cropping up in my work:

1. *Boredom*: This can result from a mutual avoidance of aggressive or competitive feelings.

   The attempt to keep such feelings at a distance may lead to an absence of emotional contact. A similar reaction can arise from discomfort with affectionate or erotic feelings on the part of the member or worker or both. Being treated like a thing or object for periods of time by the group can also reduce involvement and stimulate boredom.

2. *Sleep*: This has similar origins. It may also represent an attempt to 'kill' or eliminate the worker or a particular member, or keep the group at a distance and protect oneself from intimacy. Sleepiness and profound inertia may also be the group's way of showing an unempathic or demanding worker the power of the unconscious and the difficulty in moving faster.

   The use of stories like 'Sleeping Beauty' or 'Snow White' can be helpful in generating a context for exploration and inquiry.

3. *Devaluing*: Sometimes workers can find that they have disparaging, contemptuous or derogatory thoughts and feelings about members of the group. This may indicate that the group has projected a devalued self-image onto the worker, who has responded by devaluing the group in turn, instead of thinking about what has happened and using it to open up the aggressive or inadequate feelings.

4. *Zealousness*: Workers may behave in a zealous or over-dedicated way with the group. Extending the session time, being unusually active, caring, or committed indicates that the

worker is behaving under the influence of demanding or ideal-izing projections. Alternatively, the group may split off and project their inadequacy, dependency, fear and vulnerability onto the worker, evoking in him heroic efforts to protect him-self against these uncomfortable feelings by his zealous activity. As always, think about what might be happening and discuss with the group.

5. *Guilt*: Workers may feel guilt that they do not care enough about the group or are not skilled enough or are not doing enough to help.

   This guilt may defend against strong negative and angry feel-ings about the group being slow or difficult. It is important for the worker to acknowledge this anger to himself in order to deal with its source, which may in fact be the group's own projected aggression. In this way the worker's counter-transference anger can be used to help the group manage their own feelings of hostility and express them appropriately, instead of acting them out by missing sessions, being late, and behaving rudely.

6. *Erotic and affectionate feelings*: It is only natural that members in a group will come to have erotic and affectionate feelings for the worker who looks after them through thick and thin, and it is only natural for a worker to have erotic and affectionate feelings when members esteem them. It can be tempting to accept such feelings as one's due instead of using the counter-transference feelings to empathize with how deeply attached the group members wish to be and with how frustrating it must be not to have such desires totally gratified. Other workers may become so threatened by these feelings that they may recoil and withdraw, become unempathic and distant. Such workers need help to understand and permit their loving feelings in order to stay engaged and helpful to their group.

Review

- In order to work more intensively with group experience, the leader must learn how to focus and contexualize.
- Focusing is about observing what is happening. Contextual-izing is about making sense of what is happening.
- The worker represents an investigative attitude and an ethic of exploration and inquiry.

- There are a number of contexts in a group which correspond to different types of preoccupation.
- The worker can use his own subjective experience of the group to focus on what is happening and generate appropriate contexts.

Chapter 12

Working more synthetically with the group

To the casual observer looking in on the group it appears that a collection of people are interacting, talking, experiencing, and being with each other quite spontaneously. This is true of course, but the more practised observer would see other things occurring. Such an observer would see a spectrum of variegated human preoccupations, concerns, and aspirations refracted through the prism of the group modality.

I have already indicated something of the spectrum of the human soul in my discussion about different contexts for understanding group behaviour and dynamics, but now I want to assert some key principles and concepts which will enable us to explore the spectrum further.

Key principles

Synthesis

Synthesis means the coming together or combining of parts to make a higher-level whole. It is the primary principle which informs the practice of the creative groupworker.[1]

You have probably seen and handled the Russian babushka doll which reveals a tiered series of dolls all enfolded inside one large doll.

This is a lovely analogue for a central paradox about groupwork which revolves around the idea of unity and diversity: that groupwork is really about a process which involves multiplicity and union. The group itself is one, but is composed of many members who come together to create an experience which would otherwise be unavailable to a singleton. Group experience is what is felt and lived by the members at any one time but is also pluri-dimensional and composed of many levels. For ease of identification and to enable effective interventions, I suggested that there were five levels or contexts which would make group and individual behaviour comprehensible:

- Explicit context
- Transference context
- Projection context
- Somatic context
- Archetypal context

These contexts are personal and shared, conscious and unconscious, intra-psychic, interpersonal, and transpersonal or archetypal aspects and qualities of the human being. They are inter-penetrating and mutually and reciprocally influencing but are fundamentally the expression of this principle of synthesis – the dynamic towards wholeness and emergence out of lower-order and more primitive functioning.

In other words, groupwork is a synthetic activity which includes all the expressions and preoccupations, manifestations and associations of the human being, and shapes and links them powerfully and purposefully into an order, harmony, and beauty which elevates and transforms both the individual and the group.

Identity and the Self

Identity is what marks us out and stamps us as a particular and unique individual. Again there is this paradox of multiplicity and union; we are aware of many aspects and sides to ourselves; we live in many and sometimes contradictory worlds – and yet there is a enduring sense of being a person, of having a core identity or essential self.

Having an essential self means that the Self is the essential identity and so the five contexts of experience which we have been looking at are simply ways of describing certain attributes and preoccupations of the Self. The Self that I am:

- Has a body
- Has a psychology
- Is a social being
- Is preoccupied with existential, ethical, and transcendental questions

This knowledge is of profound importance for the groupworker, because it makes comprehensible the behaviour of a group in certain circumstances by illuminating the spectrum of motivations and concerns of its members and indicating how group membership serves the needs of the individual.

As we saw in Chapter 3, when discussing Maslow's contribution to our understanding of the motivational impulses in the person, the ultimate need is for Self-actualization – to become everything that one is capable of – although one also has various other needs at varying times. Indeed, the multiplicity of groups exist in order to help individuals deal with different levels of need and so, from a synthetic perspective different models and schools, are not contradictory but complementary. But irrespective of whatever purpose the group has been set up to achieve, one is dealing with whole human beings, and the effective group is one which achieves its goal by appropriately embracing the whole human being.

The effective group fosters a deepening sense of identity and awareness in its members of their essential Self by paying attention to and focusing on:

A psychophysical context:	Embodiment – being related to a particular body and environment – what we have called the somatic context
A psychological context:	Subjective experience – consciousness, a sense of agency and intention. Unconsciousness – a sense that some of our experience and responses emanate from feelings deep within ourselves of which we may be hardly aware – the transference and projection contexts

| A psychosocial context: | Relationship – intrinsic involvement in a social medium of meanings, customs, politics, and culture – the explicit context |
| A psychospiritual context: | Self-awareness, purpose, values, ethics, meaning, intuition, creativity, imagination, The archetypal context |

This spectrum of concerns and preoccupations is complicated by the fact that a particular individual or group may generally live and operate in one of these contexts but can experience them all. Most groups, in fact, are set up to explore one of these contexts in detail but it is clear that a person's identity shifts constantly throughout the spectrum and this will intrude on the group. The synthetic groupworker must learn to recognize when these contexts are infusing and permeating the group, and how to manage them in order to assist the group move towards its objective. We will turn to this task shortly.

Bifocal vision

Bifocal vision simply means the worker's capacity to see through the surface manifestations of group and individual behaviour and circumstances to the underlying impulse of Self towards wholeness and emergence.

Human development can be viewed as a series of expansions of identity. The core identity is that of Self, and the process is of self becoming its Self – moving from unconsciousness through consciousness to Self-consciousness or awareness or oneself as an autonomous being capable of intentionality and choice.

The function of the group is to act as an incubator and transformer of human consciousness, and the role of the groupworker is to position himself at the appropriate level in the group in order to facilitate the emergence of the next stage of individual and group growth.

Individuals and groups do not grow and develop in a steady process. Growth can be arrested for all sorts of reasons and on occasions groups may seem to regress or revert to earlier stages, patterns, or modes of functioning. This is very common. How often has one heard friends or colleagues speak about their experience of 'one step forward and two steps backward', or had such an experience oneself.

When faced with a challenge or invitation to live and respond in a new way people frequently regress to older and no longer helpful ways of behaving. They may not yet have the necessary skills or confidence and may need to access and rework earlier phases and levels of development in order to facilitate reorganization of their personality along new lines or in new patterns.

It is important for the worker to understand and manage behaviour in the group which appears regressive, because it may herald the dawn of an expansion in identity and self-knowledge and provide opportunities for individual and group development. The synthetic groupworker views regression in the group not as something to be eliminated but as presenting a possibility for growth and for the emergence of the essential Self. What enables the worker to reframe regressive behaviour and reach for its emergent potential is the worker's capacity to practise bifocal vision.

Bifocal vision enables the worker to view the group as:

• A place of formation:	Identity and self-awareness
• A place of reformation:	Correction, assistance with arrested or malformed identity
• A place of transformation:	Awakening the Self, evoking compassion, developing a sense of purpose and service

Bifocal vision enables the worker to discriminate between behaviour which is regressive and behaviour which is more obviously emergent:

Regressive behaviour	Emergent behaviour
1 Cannot tolerate difference or opposition	Accepts difference and opposition
2 Emphasizes group and mass at expense of individual	Emphasizes right relations between individuals and group

3 Compels and imposes	Negotiates and dialogues
4 Automatic, instinctual	Choice, autonomous
5 Dependent, over-reliant on authority	Self-reliant, co-operative
6 Rivalrous, selfish, violent, suspicious, contemptuous	Generative, altruistic, committed to service, compassionate
7 Façades and images	Authentic and genuine
8 Exclusive, separative, withdrawn, elitist	Inclusive, mutual, reciprocal, shares and contributes
9 Sub-groupings, factionalism, tribal, cults	Co-operative view, holistic, community
10 Ruthless, lacks conscience, rebellious, flouts rules	Moral, ethical, growing awareness of social, political issues which affect group life

The will

The will is the direct expression and capacity of an individual to function freely according to his own intrinsic nature rather than under the compulsion of external forces. A conscious act of will is one of the most powerful ways of experiencing oneself as a self-directing being, a free and responsible agent. This involves not being swept up in powerful drives, impulses, attachments, and emotions but developing the capacity to regulate and direct oneself and initiate action rather than submitting passively to it.[2]

The function of the will is to direct and choose. I am not talking here about the Victorian idea of will-power with its connotations of superior force and imposition from above or outside. This is vital for the synthetic groupworker to grasp, because it makes all the difference in terms of the quality of group experience and the kind of ethic which informs the practice of groupwork.

The concept of will is intimately linked with moral and ethical questions and the formation of a value system which guides behaviour. One of the essential features which separates the human from other life forms is the human's capacity for rational judgement and planning based on an ability to articulate values and to conduct one's life on the basis of some system of ethical principles. This intentionality and moral agency is the core of human identity and a central pursuit of the groupworker.

The worker's constant care is to enable group members to develop mutually agreed, self-generated, and internalized controls and values rather than acquiescing to externally asserted norms and values. From this perspective the group serves the process of individuation – becoming oneself – and the individual, by choosing group membership as a means of expressing and actualizing himself, through belonging to and relating to others, finds himself inevitably in the service of the group goals.

The group moves closer to the ideal of community as autonomous individuals now act out their own will and initiative to come together to express and fulfil their purpose. This invariably involves members re-choosing to be in the group. Power and authority is no longer simply invested in the leader but is a function and right of membership and the inner experience of the individual. You can see that the groupworker seeks every opportunity to activate and foster the members' will and cultivate the intentional and moral capacity of the individual and the group. This allows the worker to include a range of psychosocial, cultural, political, existential, and ethical concerns that many other groupwork models would exclude, reduce, or pathologize.

A definition of synthetic groupwork

Synthetic groupwork refers to the conscious, disciplined, and systematic use of knowledge about the known processes, manifestations, and goals of human behaviour, interaction, and aspiration, in order to intervene in an informed way or promote a desired objective in a group setting. Synthetic groupwork is a helping process designed to correspond to specific instances of individual and group need, based on a view of humans whose core project is expanding their identity by awakening the Self, leading to Self realization and Self actualization.

Let's turn now to consider this spectrum in practice.

Working with the psychophysical dimension of the group

Embodiment is absolutely central to being a person. The body is the vehicle for existing and being in the world and a precious instrument of experience and action. Embodiment also has a psychological and social dimension, because the body is essential as:

- A ground for one's sense of self and perception of reality
- A vehicle for sensory awareness and emotional responses
- A means of self-expression
- A medium for communication and contact

The body is simply a way of being an incarnate self, and it is the self in the body which converts sensations and physiological phenomena into significant psychological experience and meaning. Important in this is the total psychological field, current and resonant, in which the sensations are produced.

A group is a rich sensory and psychological field because of the presence of other people and the potential to be publicly shamed, attacked, blamed or affirmed, touched, contacted, and embraced. Add to this environment such factors as spaces which are large, small, private, public, intimate, boring, stressful; changes in scale, lighting, temperature, noise, smells; activities which are verbal, physical, emotional, fast and slow paced, messy and clean – and you can well understand how being in a group with other people can generate somatic and emotional responses.

Groups can amplify and magnify these responses cybernetically, which is why people sometimes avoid or dread groups because of their fears of regression. Group membership involves some loosening of the usual boundaries of the self in order to participate, and in beginning groups of relative strangers or times of heightened emotion this frequently generates feelings of contagion and invasion accompanied by varying degrees of depersonalization or de-individuation. This is why groups sometimes feel 'cold' or anxious, and the worker may use 'icebreakers', 'warm-ups', and 'contact games'.

Of course, temporary loss or suspension of personality can also be a pleasant, even transcendent, feeling and connect us to an ecstatic or tribal and herd experience which may be actively sought out, as when one goes to a rave or pop concert or a football match and the mass experience is spontaneous and uplifting, instinctual and exhilarating.

Here are some manifestations of the psychophysical dimension of the group:

Members report the following:	The worker is aware of:
• Heart thumping	• Cold/frozen silences
• Sweaty palms	• Stammering
• Dry mouth	• Chattering/repetitiveness
• Butterflies in stomach	• Hysterical laughter
• Difficulty in thinking	• Impulsive behaviour
• Stomatic/hypochondriacal symptoms	• Greed/aggression/ vandalism
• Pains/aches/nausea/ headaches	• Sleepiness, boredom
• Back tension	• Blushing/embarrassment/ shame
• Feelings of deadness/ woodenness	
• The group/other/activity is making me feel this way/ putting something into me	

The psychophysical quality of group experience means that it is hard to think about and hard to verbalize.

The mindlessness, powerful sensations, and emotions churned up are initially very frightening and the group is prone to impulsive behaviour and acting out. In order to manage such discharges, the worker may decide to think and speak for the group.

Example

It was the second session of a personal development group and the members seemed to take turns to complain about the hardness of the chairs, the coldness of the room, the noise outside the room, their anxiety about my unnerving silence, difficulty speaking, rising panic. Some members would leave their seat, pace around the room, go to the window, go to the toilet, drum their fingers, and tap their feet.

Intervention: I decided to come in as people were getting very anxious, and said that beginnings were often difficult and even traumatic for some people. The birth of a group, like that of an individual, might be such a traumatic experience and one that was hard to bear. I suggested that it might be helpful to view their physical experiences as their way of handling and communicating the discomfort of coming into being as a group.

My intention was to:

- Acknowledge the physicality of the members' early experience of the group
- Normalize this
- Contextualize the material by using the physical metaphor of birth
- Reformulate the physical experience as the basis for reflection, group discussion, and interaction

---

In other situations the worker may 'contain' the psychophysical experience in the group. This means that the worker makes a space inside himself where he can think about the process of the group's anxieties. Containing the group's psychophysical tension and anxiety when the group is prone to energy discharge and acting out is demanding, and involves the worker's utilizing the counter-transference capacity and skills which we looked at earlier. The worker is empathetically and non-verbally modelling a way of dealing with anxiety which members intuitively relate to and can recognize as different from those occasions when the worker is inattentive, absent, or bored. The template for this is the relaxed and non-anxious mother, of pre-verbal experience.

The important thing to remember when confronted by psycho-physical phenomena and somatizing in the group is not to ignore it but to begin to think about what the group is communicating through this early identity. Re-read the earlier section on the worker's use of self, and try to internalize this mode of thinking and behaving in your group.

Working with the psychological dimension of the group

Each individual in the group has their own idiosyncratic way of being in the world and making sense of that experience. The highly subjective nature of members' perception and modes of relating means that the group process is often highly charged with emotions – anxiety-producing, contradictory, and changeable – and that the group process in turn colours and permeates members' responses. Helping people understand what goes into their subjective experience of an event or phenomenon, clarifying how their response differs or radically diverges from others' experience, and creatively managing the dissonance is an important and ongoing activity for the worker. Helping people think psychologically rather than concretely and literally is vital if the group is learning to work with and manage its own process.

Teaching members to work psychologically involves coaching them to:

- See and identify patterns, connections, recurring themes/motifs
- Pause, reflect, ponder, muse, wonder
- Think imaginatively, symbolically
- Avoid concrete and literal thought
- Include feelings and emotions
- Include intuitions
- Include somatic communication
- Bridge between inner and outer worlds of experience
- Become familiar with the idea of unconscious motives
- Recognize the contribution of childhood experience to personality formation
- Become familiar with ideas of repetition and re-enactment of habitual interaction sets
- Recognize defensive reactions and patterns

Re-read the section on page 233 outlining the worker's cultivation of the investigative attitude in the group, and the section on page 241 which gives detailed advice on how to employ the worker's subjective experience to work more intensively with the group. This will confirm what I mean about working more psychologically.

Working with defensive reactions in the group

Defence mechanisms and reactions are attempted 'solutions' to intra-psychic and interpersonal conflicts. They are ways of disguising and distorting shameful, painful, or hidden feelings and desires from oneself and others. The checklists on pages 89–90, 105–106 and 147 will give you an idea of how defences manifest in groups.

Defensive reactions are easily stimulated in the group, and must be dealt with sensitively if change is to occur.

Some group workers take the position that defences are 'enemies' which must be overcome, but I believe this to be an archaic and mistaken view, in that to perceive defences thus is to break empathy with the group in a fundamental way and to reinforce the very behaviour which you wish to see changed. The worker's goal is to help group members move from rigid and debilitating ways of behaving to more flexible and appropriate forms of interaction.

Defensive activity in the group originates from three sources:

1   *Defences in the individual member*: There are a myriad of defences in which individuals will engage, ranging from silence to self-absorption, detachment, cynicism, fault finding, or aggression – anything that will alter the tone, level, or direction of group experience away from intimacy and vulnerability. Watch out for recurrent themes and repetitive situations which indicate the presence of anxiety and the attempt to defend against it.

    The nature of groupwork requires individuals to participate actively if it is to work, and such close proximity can cause anxiety for individuals. Some members will respond with exaggerated independence or feel compelled to be rebellious and destructive. Others may exhibit inappropriate dependence on the leader or be self-harmful.

    Managing such reactions involves making explicit the underlying aggression and fear of contact while endeavouring to develop the capacity for concern, mutuality, and interdependence in the group.

2   *Defences of the group as a whole*: Defensive activity may emerge as a response to the needs of the whole group. Re-read the example on page 231 which shows how the existing group

responded anxiously and defensively to the introduction of new members. You can see how the group is organizing and coping with its anxiety by being attentive to events and phenomena which are significant and carry meaning and anxiety for the collective membership, such as:

- The entry of new members
- The departure of senior members
- Holiday breaks
- Change of venue/time/frequency
- The worker's illness or pregnancy
- The termination of the group
- External events – the Dunblane massacre, the Omagh bomb, Kosovo, etc.

3   *Defences arising from the worker's counter-transference*: The combined weight of members' expectations, behaviour, and anxiety can exert enormous pressure on a worker psychologically. This regressive pull can tax even the most experienced groupworker and undermine objectivity and empathy. When the worker is a novice or is undergoing personal stress, it can happen that the worker withdraws emotionally and avoids or defends against the full impact of the group process. To some degree this is inevitable at some time in every group. See the example given on page 245, where I allowed things to run on inappropriately in the group because I was unwilling to experience myself or present as the final authority.

The defences arise from four underlying fears and anxieties which deter members from reaching out to each other emotionally, and excite protective action:

1 Fear of impulsivity – being flooded or overwhelmed by instincts and emotions leads to behaviour which emphasizes control and avoidance.
2 Fear of abandonment may provoke exaggerated independence as a form of denial, or it may bring out its opposite – clinging and dependent behaviour and phobic responses.

3 Fear of merging or being taken over or engulfed may incite suspicious and hostile behaviour and inappropriate self-reliance.

4 Fear of vulnerability – being hurt, humiliated, or revealed as inadequate can generate grandiosity, expressions of disdain and contempt, or lofty and isolated behaviour

The worker should focus on each member's characteristic style of relating in order to help that person understand the effect and consequences of that style. By examining the biographical events and current triggers in the group, members can come to understand what led up the need to behave so defensively and gradually learn to acquire more appropriate and better ways of protecting and asserting themselves.

Try to demonstrate how the individual or group is behaving and give examples which are difficult to refute. Clarify the motives of the defensive behaviour by identifying the fear which drives it. Determine what is triggering the behaviour now and whether it is an old memory or situation, or a current event which usually can be more easily dealt with.

Working with transference reactions in the group

The presence of others is a powerful stimulant and can enhance the possibility of exposing a variety of relationships and broaden the context in which members' less healthy interactions can be examined.

Groups can promote a situation of regression and provide opportunities for the development of parental transferences to the worker and sibling transferences to peers. The example given on page 245 shows these vertical and horizontal transferences quite clearly, so you might wish to re-read this vignette.

It is essential that you understand that transference reactions occur frequently in groups and that they radically influence the nature of group behaviour. Groupworkers who ignore or misunderstand transference manifestation may seriously misunderstand some transactions and confuse rather than guide the group members.

Recognizing transference reactions

Transference can be simply defined as the experiencing and manifestation of feelings, behaviours, attitudes, fantasies, and defences
by one person towards another in the present which do not fit that
person but are repetitions of reactions and behaviours originating in
relation to significant persons in childhood. So a group member
may respond to the worker in the sorts of ways in which they
responded to a parent in childhood – looking for help, wanting
admiration, rebelling against the rules. Or they may respond to
peers in the group as if they were siblings – competing for the
worker's attention, bullying each other, creating gangs and sub-
groups. You can be sure that transference is occurring when you
observe behaviour which is:

- Inappropriate/out of context
- Repetitious, recurring, cyclical
- Intense/over the top
- Ambivalent
- Tenacious, resistant to explanation

Always give yourself time to observe how members relate to and
use each other, how they relate to and use you, and reflect upon
your own feelings and process. Gradually you will become aware of
how the past is being repeated in the present and enshrouding new
possibilities with a sort of archaic psychological cling-film.

Here are three tips:

Look for behaviour	
A *at a group level* • Dependent behaviour aimed at eliciting protection/security from all-powerful leader • Group is experienced as a skin or body; breast or like mother	B *at an individual level* • Repetitive and reliant questioning • Preoccupation with procedures/tasks • Silence/chattering/ superficiality

- Fight–flight behaviour aimed at helping group gain security by battle or escape
- Formation of sub-groups/gangs which contain safe/unsafe desired, feared parts of member's self

- Withdrawal/self-sufficiency
- Hovering/hesitation, sitting on the fence
- Clinging/over-dependent behaviour
- Exhibitionism, boasting/vandalism/aggression/bullying, expressions of contempt or indifference
- Absenteeism, lateness, refusal to join in
- Unwillingness to trust/fear of vulnerability/being taken over

Listen to themes in members' discussion	
A *People and relationship themes and quality of interaction* • Stories and narratives about activity or intent of employers/bosses, leaders, politicians/authority figures, shopworkers/service workers • Stories about work colleagues/team mates/friends/partners, neighbours	*Implicit message for worker/peers* • Worker is parental figure who is abusive, interfering, exploitative, deceitful, or, alternatively, loving, helpful, generous, committed, zealous, reliable • Group peers are siblings who are rivals, envious, hostile, belligerent, greedy, deceitful, or, alternatively, loving, generous, compassionate, indispensable

B *Places and locations and their qualities*	
• Stories about busy bus/rail/ tube stations; dentist's/ doctor's waiting room, or descriptions of peaceful/ distracting or desired or feared rural/urban/ seaside/mountain settings	• References to quality of group experience, interaction, communication or quality of worker's attention and empathy. May also indicate family re-enactments triggered off by current participation

How things work and don't work	
• Stories about broken cars/ washing machines, dishwashers/leaking pipes/ blocked drains, accounts of unsuccessful/winning athletic/sports performances, efficient or poorly performing, business/government/ health service	• Reference to how well group opportunity or the worker is functioning or malfunctioning may indicate family re-enactments or early group/ school/work/church experiences or current membership of external groups

I could give many more examples but I think that you can see how important it is to reflect upon the individual or group behaviour and story and consider the underlying subtext as a communication about transference preoccupations concerning the worker or the other members. Ask yourself: who is the person who is speaking now – adult, adolescent, child? What are they saying about their experience of the group, other members, the worker? What family scenario, sibling or parental relationship is being re-enacted now?

If it appears that the group or individual interaction is immature or inappropriate or repetitious, then you can be sure that you are witnessing transference behaviour. My own approach to dealing with transference in the group is based on identifying whether it is best to intervene at the level of the group as a whole or draw attention to interpersonal or individual patterns and configurations.

Consider the presenting material and assess the group members' ability to examine their functioning in the group, and intervene at the level that will best engage them.

This may mean emphasizing the individual's life and examining the person's biography and character formation for clues as to their typical defences, problem-solving techniques, and ways of regarding and relating to themselves. The next level of intervention is the interpersonal, which points out rational styles and considers what internalized conflicts with siblings, peers, and authority figures is being replayed in the here-and-now interpersonal field. On the collective level, group-as-a-whole dynamics can be explored, illuminating early mother–infant relations as well as including valuable information about the operation of group norms, values, assumptions, and restrictions.

Try to gather evidence and examples of repetitive and therefore irrefutable patterns which you can use to demonstrate the manifestation of transference phenomena. Clarify just what it is about the worker or another member which triggers associations and feelings with significant people and episodes from the past. Explore the feelings and fantasies involved in the transference reaction and try to make a link with the surface interactions and the underlying causes. In this way you can make sense of the transference and help the individual and the group understand what is going on. You will probably have to repeat this activity many times before the transference behaviour will be modified, so don't worry if it recurs.

These patterns were learned a long time ago and take a long time to go away. The important thing is to establish and promote in your group a culture of inquiry and curiosity which engages members in a routine and ongoing examination of their behaviour and motives.

Working with the psychosocial dimension of the group

The idea of a psychosocial dimension in the group is based on the notion that there is an interactional synchrony between the essential self and the relational and social-cultural context in which it emerges, and that this intertwining of self and social context is replicated in the group. The groupworker needs to be alert to phenomena and preoccupations which reflect individual and group concerns with important and relevant social and political issues and which can serve the development of the group as a sensitive and responsive instrument for the expansion of individual identity and conscience.

Individual identity is a synthesis of personal experiences and attitudes and social arrangements and institutions. Identity and personhood are socially and culturally organized by access to and experience of these behaviours, practices, and systems:

- Family experiences
- Child-rearing practices
- Kinship systems and social class
- Educational institutions
- Religious upbringing
- Political affiliations
- Gender, sexual identity, sexism
- Marriage and relationship
- Racial and ethnic origins and identity
- Economic systems, markets
- Labour, relations, employment, joblessness
- Law, policing, military
- Art, culture, media
- Leisure, entertainment
- Technology, science, medicine
- Ecology, environmental issues
- National and international politics
- Catastrophe, war, terrorism

Since these activities are contained within the individual in the forms of habits, attitudes, and experience, it is inevitable that at times the group will find itself having to confront issues and concerns which mirror debates or dilemmas in the wider society and which enter or permeate the group matrix. Learn to include these concerns imaginatively rather than tell yourself or the group that such issues have nothing to do with the group objective.

Stretching yourself and the group to make space for such reflection and discussion creates an ethos of inclusion and inquiry which can provide an opportunity for a sense of empowerment and engagement with the central issues of the day and, in fact, actually further the group goals – whatever they may be – through direct experiential learning, metaphor, and analogue.

Example I

The idea that the individual reflects not just a personal but also a collective and even historical identity is, not surprisingly, a daily and permanent feature of my work in Northern Ireland. In the Northern Ireland context there are a myriad of coded signals which are available and inculturated into the individual from birth and which communicate one's ethnic group, religious background, and likely political allegiance. One's school, address, place of work, and even one's name functions as a potent cultural signal. I recall how in one group a Protestant woman persisted in denying that a significant member for her was a Catholic by consistently calling him Donald when his name was in fact Donal and it was repeatedly pointed out to her. Unconsciously, she had to make him a cultural partner by adjusting the one letter of his name before she could allow him to mean anything to her.

Only as she was able to become aware of this previously unconscious and now unwanted prejudice towards Catholics could she, and subsequently the group, begin to explore how a sheltered and exclusive upbringing might adversely affect a person in many other ways and prevent groups of people from different religious and cultural backgrounds relating honestly and intimately with each other.

Usually these sorts of cultural signifiers and codes are well understood and rarely made explicit. Indeed, one of the recurring difficulties of my work with groups in this type of sociopolitical context has been exposing the effects and consequences of such implicit and subliminal communication, and making plain the profound denial caused by the fear that the destructive fantasies underpinning much of this communication will invade the group and become 'reality'. Group members will frequently go to great lengths to ensure that the internal cohesion of the group is not threatened by the daily catalogue of terror or grievance in the wider society, or their own role in that society. Despite their best efforts, however, unconscious formations that originate not in individual repression but as expressions of social and cultural conditioning constantly reveal themselves in the group.

Example 2

In the early stages of another group a man came to the session wearing a remembrance poppy. Now, this simple act of remembrance to the dead of two world wars has a particular resonance in Northern Ireland. Few Catholics would wear this poppy. It is associated with certain Protestant and British loyalties and as such could be construed by some as a declaration in favour of the political union with Westminster and therefore anti-nationalist. This member was one of three Protestants in the group, which contained three Catholics and two of other denominations. No one else wore a poppy, and it was not referred to although we were all aware of its significance.

As the session unfolded, two of the Catholic members in this hitherto placid group became increasingly angry with me, condemning me for routinely saying little except to demand something more from them. Gradually other members joined in, criticizing me for wearing a suit which made them feel that I was like an oppressive authority, and commenting on the tension I caused in the group by my unhelpful presence.

In a different culture I might have understood the criticism of me as relating to the beginning anxieties of members and their angry perception of me as a depriving and authoritative parent, and, I would have intervened accordingly. However, in a Northern Irish context, an intervention based solely on this insight would have missed the cultural subtext, It was also clear that there was a deep displacement onto me of anger which was really directed at the member who was perceived to distinguish himself by his dress – the wearing of a poppy – as a representative of a hated political authority and rival group.

It was not possible to engage him or the group in those early days in an open discussion of the themes of symbols, allegiances, enemies, and rivalries because of the group's fear that such discussion would invite the possibility of 'war' in the group. My intervention was taken up in part – the political dimension being dropped quickly. But it did not simply disappear. A dimension of members' lives had been acknowledged and an ethos of inquiry had been introduced. As the group developed there was a growing interest in political and cultural differences, and one year later, when the same man wore his poppy to the session, there was a vigorous exchange of political views which was authentic and led to a more mature and ongoing exploration of what it was like to live and interact in a polarized society.

Since 1989 I have been working on a regular basis in England with supervision groups, experiential learning groups, and teaching groups, which include a wide range of ages, sexual orientations, and ethnic and racial backgrounds, and I have found these groups to be identically affected by and resonating to events and issues in their particular sociopolitical context. At various times I have found that I need to include members' concerns or make references to the dominant issues of the day in order to facilitate a group preoccupied with an external event, or to illustrate how some piece of group process is proceeding along the lines of some structural issue in the wider society.

Example 3

I recall working with a large group of about eighty student psychotherapists in London shortly after the Dunblane massacre, in which a deranged gunman murdered a number of children and their teacher in their school in 1997. My group of students felt shocked and numbed by the tragedy, and experienced a deep sense of helplessness and anxiety that it was impossible to prevent such a thing happening. As students and parents themselves, they felt a deep bond of empathy and affinity with the murdered children and their bereaved parents.

The whole two-hour session was taken up with the group members sensitively and profoundly exploring a whole range of issues and dilemmas to do with living and working in a modern society in which such random and alienated actions occurred. This poignant and sorrowful discussion was a mirror of the same discussion taking place in the wider society, in the media, in workplaces and social meeting points. The group came to no conclusions, of course, but a gathering of some eighty people were enabled to speak about how they were experiencing a major national trauma, and reflect upon and struggle with the sorts of questions and dilemmas it raised for them as members of that society.

I could give innumerable examples similar to this of how the social and cultural context permeates the group and affects members' psychology and relationships.

Here are a few illustrations of how certain events impinged upon and stirred up issues in some of my groups:

Social/cultural/political issues	Members' preoccupations
• Gulf War/Bosnian War/ Kosovo/Canary Wharf bombing/IRA terrorism	• National identify; fears of being member of racial or ethnic minority; how groups manage difference, aggression, conflict
• Lowering of age of homosexual consent	• Sexual orientation, homophobia, relations between men and women
• Stephen Lawrence case	• Racial harassment, discrimination of Irish, Blacks, Jews, family experiences of Holocaust, relations with authority, police, teachers, one's internal authority
• Technological/scientific/ medical advances, cloning, geno-programme, spare-part surgery	• Fears of Big Brother, helplessness, uncertainty about authority and big business, alienation, worries about not being consulted, illness, ageing, death
• Environmental, ecological disasters/catastrophes, BSE beef crisis, food scares	• Anger about poor responses by authority, lack of empathy, compassion, concern about corporate greed, indifference, impotence, helplessness
• Millennium issues	• How and what to celebrate/remember, secular versus sacred, hopes/fears for future, new beginnings, rituals

This is a brief sample of some of the social issues that have engrossed my groups and the types of discussion which ensued. You can see from the members' preoccupations that there is a correlation between their public and personal response to the issues. Members have emotional and political responses to events and this is the very stuff of group membership and experience. The core issues centre on what it means to be a person in a social world – with the fears, dreads, hopes, and longings this raises. Members have to struggle with the essential group dilemma I described on page 239: how to get close but not too close and how be separate but not too separate:

- What makes people similar to and different from each other?
- What rights and responsibiities do people have regarding each other?
- What is the relationship between the individual and the group?
- What is the nature of society/community?
- How do groups manage disagreements and conflicts?
- How should a group best organize itself?

Utilizing psychosocial material in the group

Acknowledging the reality of the concerns

Sometimes it can be an indication of emotional well-being and civic responsibility if an individual or a group raises a particular issue. It can indicate a reasonable and appropriate relation with reality and a healthy response to one's actual environment or life circumstances. It would be very worrying to me, for example, if none of my groups which met the week following the Omagh bomb explosion in August 1998 had spoken about their shock and horror at an atrocity which killed so many people and appalled the world. What members in these groups needed was an opportunity to grieve collectively and to experience the comfort and solidarity of being in the presence of other people who felt exactly as they did.

In other situations – for instance, if a group member or relative has had a serious illness or surgery – their experience of the

National Health Service may provoke discussion about the merits and demerits of this system and raise issues about the commitment of political parties to the service. To talk about cuts, economies, and waiting lists may raise legitimate questions about personal values and principles and values in society.

The experience of members or their relatives of police or security forces may reflect actual injustice or discrimination and harassment; this may require space in the group for the reality to be acknowledged that sometimes authority can be oppressive and the law can be an ass. Similarly, individual stories about sexual or gender discrimination at work, accounts of homophobic prejudice and even assault, and racial discrimination and bullying need to be honoured and validated if the group is to prove its worth as a sanctuary and a place where things can be different.

Individuals come to groups with a whole range of concerns and anxieties about what is happening in science and genetics and the Internet, with ecological and environmental fears, worries about world debt and ownership of the media, and a myriad of other social, cultural, and political issues. It is important that the group-worker straightforwardly acknowledge and affirm the reality of these preoccupations as a sign of mature and civic responsibility, and endeavours to make the group a place where such discussion contributes to the cohesion and relevance of the group experience in its members' lives.

A fundamental task of any group is to raise members' consciousness of particular issues of concern to them, so including the reality of the world in which members live contributes greatly to their capacity to reflect deeply on the wider social meaning of their problems and struggles.

Opening up the psychological and symbolic level of the material

Often psychosocial events can be used by individuals and groups to communicate some internal and unconscious worries or fears. In the case of the Omagh bomb, members of my groups continued to speak about the atrocity for a very long time after the event. In some cases people spoke about their sense of evil or hopelessness that the peace process could stay on track and their fears of societal collapse. Now, this was a real danger, since terrorism aims to strike at people's belief and trust that authority can look after them by savagely undercutting the basis of hope and trust in security and civic protection, but this attack seemed for many to arouse a deeper sense of personal responsibility and culpability.

Members reported feelings of guilt that they had survived when so many had randomly died, a sense of impotence and helplessness to effect change, and a belief that somehow they had contributed to the problem over the years by not more actively renouncing violent groups and politics.

This is a common experience of witnesses and bystanders to traumatic events and catastrophes, both man-made and natural; it requires the groupworker to tune into members' distress sensitively and empathically in order to gauge how an external event may mirror some internal anxiety or re-awaken some long-dormant dread and worry.

In other situations individuals and groups may use social or cultural issues to protect or defend themselves from the effects of more immediate and personal concerns. The preoccupations with and anger about the state of the Health Service or the government's commitment may, in reality, distract from the individual's personal engagement with their own ageing or illness, or divert the group from having to encounter the pain of finiteness and limitation when struggling to help members with those all too intractable problems.

Similarly, the sense of injustice and experience of victimization reported by members may, in addition to reality factors, contain projections of their own internal bully and victim interactions and unresolved grandiosity, and defend against feelings of inferiority and worthlessness. This may manifest as an exaggerated, even belligerent, advocacy of gay rights, environmental concerns, animal rights, and a host of other assertions. It is important to explore sensitively the underlying feelings of hostility and fears of persecution if the manifest concerns for social justice and fairness are to be given an appropriate and rightful place.

External social events may mirror the group's perception of its own internal arrangements, customs, and experiences. Most group leaders at some point have been compared to Adolf Hitler or Saddam Hussein, and one can readily see the transference projections of the bad father and the cruel, dictatorial group leader who makes demands and imposes rules on the membership. The group's interest in recent political changes in Eastern Europe, with the demise of communism, the fall of the Berlin Wall, and all the other demographic consequences, may reflect the members' implicit or unconscious longing for more power in the group and a wish to 'overthrow' the leader and usher in a fantasized era of participation and ownership. The important point to remember is that the reference to social and cultural issues may be a psychosocial metaphor or analogue for the individual or group's preoccupation with its own internal state of mind; the groupworker's difficult task is to determine when the reference is reality-based and when it reflects a deeper concern.

Here are some questions to ask when considering psychosocial material:

- What are the social/cultural/political themes in the group?
- Are they current in the external world?
- What currently is happening in the external world?
- How is it impacting on the group?
- How much of the individual/group concern is objective?
- Can I determine subjective elements?
- Why is this theme being discussed now?
- How does it serve the individual/group?
- How is this social theme a metaphor for member–leader interactions?
- Does it represent member–member interactions?
- Does it represent internal configurations within the member?
- Does it represent member/group history/biography?
- What is trying to emerge through this discussion?
- Is there an existential concern here?
- Is there an archetypal/mythic pattern being repeated?
- Does this discussion illuminate values and principles?

The synthetic groupworker recognizes the reciprocal interrelationship of personal identity and social context, and endeavours to implement a climate in which members assume a responsible attitude towards the individual, their group, and society, bearing in mind the difficulties and dilemmas involved in interacting and relating to others. The group is a microcosm of the larger collective, and by including and encouraging a psychosocial consciousness in members, the worker enables each person to participate in society and contribute to social change.

Working with the psychospiritual dimension of the group

The idea of the psychospiritual refers to levels of human consciousness that are present and potentially available in all cultures with widely varying content and context. They are concerned with:

- A meaningful philosophy of life
- Creative and purposeful values
- A sense of being a moral being
- Developing our deepest sense of self and identity
- A sense of place and trustful belonging in the universe
- A relationship with a higher/power/providence/God/divine
- Renewing moments of transcendence
- A sense of the sacred/mystery/wonder/aesthetic and beauty
- A sustaining and creative world-view

The word 'psychospiritual' does not cleanly separate psychology and spirituality but indicates an interface where individuals' mental health and psychological well-being is inextricably intertwined with their spiritual experience and growth. I want at this point to distinguish and differentiate spirituality from religion, which is a specific and organized system of faith, worship, doctrine, and rituals. 'Spirituality' is a word that defies specific definition but is often used to describe the human need for meaning and value in life and the desire for relationship with a transcendent power.

Fukuyama and Sevig report spirituality as

> an innate capacity and tendency to move towards knowledge, love, meaning, hope, transcendence, connectedness and compassion. It includes one's capacity for creativity, growth and the development of a values system. Spirituality encompasses the religious, spiritual and transpersonal.[3]

Clearly, a spiritual dimension enhances personal growth and freedom by promoting a way of being and experiencing:

- Mind
- Body

- Spirit
- Relationships with other beings
- Relationships with nature
- Relationships with work and leisure
- Relationships with organizations and institutions
- Relationships with culture and a world-view
- Relationships with life

I have already indicated that these areas are of constant concern to individuals and groups, and so it follows for me that a psychospiritual perspective and emphasis is a necessary attribute and dimension of groupwork and immensely enriches and expands the opportunity and possibility of group experience and action.

The psychospiritual dimension of the group has two characteristics:

1   An emphasis on awakening the sense of essential self in each member and with facilitating the manifestations, dilemmas, and pre-occupations of this deepest self and identity.
2   An emphasis on synthesis in the group: harmonizing, integrating, and transmitting collective and interpersonal processes so as to promote an experience of caring and responsive community which endeavours to help members move towards becoming what they are most capable of.

Example:

A woman in a group had recurring difficulty in collaborating with other members around issues of mutual concern – when a new member should arrive, changing the time of the meeting to accommodate the others, meeting with the group in the forced absence of the groupworker. These and other differences occasioned a great deal of strife between her and other members in the group because it became clear that the woman often had no real objection but was disagreeing out of her biographical history. She was the eldest child and resented her siblings, whom she felt should acknowledge and submit to her priority and authority.

She came from a family which had acquired wealth and felt elevated in a poor community, but also felt insecure about this and anxious about being the object of envy.

It became clear after much discussion over many sessions that the recurring issue for this woman revolved around her difficulty of being separate but not alienated, while being an influential member but not central. These issues of belonging, autonomy, and authority opened up for her and the group important themes to do with what members could expect from each other in terms of rights and responsibilities, issues around respect, power, and privilege, and the nature and limits of self-expression and determination.

Much of the work undertaken by this member and the group involved examining the regressive aspects of this material from a psychological and therapeutic perspective. However, what characterized the psychospiritual nature of the ongoing discussion was the capacity of the participants actively and consciously to include and engage with a sense of the person as a moral being, passionately concerned with principles, ethics, and values to do with the pain and suffering of others and the obligation of social justice. In addition, simple material values and consideration of what was ultimately satisfying, were challenged and there was an awareness that self-expression and self-determination must be based on qualities of compassion and ethical considerations if they are not to be ruthless.

This was the focus of debate when the woman member decided to take a holiday during the group term in apparent contravention of the contract to attend each session. It seemed that her will and the will of the group would conflict yet again, but instead there was a sensitive dialogue in which the woman presented a case for her holiday which involved her recognizing the obligations of group membership and asking the group to recognize her autonomy. The difference in the atmosphere of the session and the quality of discussion this time was palpable, and was characterized by a sense of love and tender, authentic relatedness. The woman was willing to surrender to the group's authority and was also negotiating the nature of her identity and relationship to the whole. She was clearly exploring interdependence and connectedness, which was firmly based on her freedom and responsibility and was in no way operating from the old familial compulsions or dynamics.

The group members were flexible and responsive, and willing to encourage creative and innovative behaviour which was motivated by mutually agreed values and principles. This had implications for the group, since it meant modifying existing rules in favour of an individual but it led to an increasing tolerance of diversity and a developing sense of community because the experience of goodwill enabled them to transcend the tendencies towards cultishness and shallow homogenization which lurk in the shadows of every group.

Group rules and norms can shackle individuals and prompt unhealthy individuation and rebellion unless the group and the member can be enabled to work with and connect to the highest values – those emphasizing the dialectic between the emergent and individuating self and a responsive and self-generating community.

The key to working at psychospiritual levels in the group lies in the capacity of the worker for that bifocal vision which permits both an exploration of regressive phenomena and behaviour where necessary, while recognizing and encouraging the underlying impulse of the essential Self towards relatedness and wholeness. Both individual and group consciousness are consequently transformed and refined. The opportunity to open up the psychospiritual concerns of group members is ever present and can be initiated by individuals as well as by the worker. Here are some examples of situations and events which generated an emphasis on more universal themes in my groups:

Outside the group but affecting members
- War/acts of terrorism/assassinations/bombings/hijackings
- Natural catastrophes – earthquakes, floods, fires
- Political corruption and sleaze
- Food scares
- Medical, technological, and scientific advances

Experience inside the group
- Death of member's relative
- Illness of member
- Presence of clergy as members
- Termination of the group
- Loss of individual's purpose/vision/vocation
- Depression
- Conflict
- Ruthless and selfish behaviour
- Lack of trust
- Cynicism and scepticism

These examples and countless others can often excite in members concerns and preoccupations about:

- The capricious and random nature of life
- Existential isolation[4]
- Anxiety about death
- Fear of freedom[5]
- A loss of meaning[6]
- Awareness of finiteness/limitation/tragedy
- The presence and nature of evil
- The nature of good
- Questioning and searching for spiritual values: idealism, altruism, compassion, justice, mercy, forgiveness, faith, hope, love, peace
- The experience of grace
- The nature of intimacy and sacredness
- The difference between conflict and paradox

These sorts of concerns and questions are the cues which can be used by a sensitive worker to help individuals and groups make meaning out of their suffering and generate new and creative contexts for living. I hardly need stress that a worker does not impose a particular religious or spiritual perspective upon the group but, rather, waits and seeks to stand for and point to a larger context within which group members can locate their dilemmas and preoccupations. This larger context is archetypally derived and spiritually informed and is put forward as a resource for healing and a source of meaning.

The importance of the psychospiritual perspective is that it offers the worker the opportunity to intervene creatively and synthetically:

Repair:	The worker can help members deal with their personal wounds by working through the regressive aspects

Individuation:	The worker can help connect and align the member and group to that inherent dynamic towards wholeness within each individual. Inevitably this involves member and group building a moral and ethical ground and identity which emphasizes agency, intentionality, responsibility, choice autonomy, right relations, and one's place in the universe

The key element for the worker is to discern and discriminate where an individual or group is most identified at any one time. In order to intervene psychospiritually, the worker seeks to awaken the sense of Self at a deep level or collaborate with the emerging Self as a free and responsible agent. The question to ask is simple but profound: *Who is this person most at this moment?*

There are only a few answers possible:

> - The person most resembles an angry/hurt/manipulative child
> - The person most resembles an idealistic/rebellious/intro-verted/awkward teenager
> - The person is most preoccupied with getting their own way and satisfying their ego needs for esteem, power, privilege
> - The person most resembles a mature adult concerned with Self-realization and Self-actualization

The first three answers give a picture of what most concerns an individual or group at any one time, and indicate that the correct intervention in group process is to focus on the psychological and developmental aspects of the difficulty. The last answer paints a portrait of an individual or group engaged in existential and spiritual inquiry and growth and indicates to the worker that a psychospiritual intervention is most appropriate.

Types of psychospiritual interventions

There are many forms of intervention that arise out of a particular situation, but here are four strategies that I find myself consistently using in my groups.

1   Depending on the situation I may recount a story or parable, or make reference to a myth or fairy tale, which opens up the archetypal context. This engages imagination, wonder, mystery, and a sense of the numinous to evoke soul qualities like love, compassion, the tragic, reverence, beauty, which may require acknowledgement and experiencing if the group is to transcend and transmute its current difficulties.

2   Frequently I will ask an individual: 'What do you stand for/ What is most important to you?' This is a way of connecting a person to their highest values, and of reminding an individual who they really are and what most motivates them. Often an individual and a group need to articulate what is most essential to them but, surprisingly, many people are able to assert their core values. What is difficult for them is how personality dynamics and biography sabotage the expression of one's deepest desires.

3   It is important to engage and evoke an individual's will. Many people feel determined by their personal history and behave in compulsive ways. I try to remind individuals that they have the power of agency and the capacity for choice even in limiting situations. The exercise of choice is a personal act of creation and involves different aspects of our experience of willing. With some groups and individuals this may require an exploration of the role of purpose and vision as a first step in the act of will.

It may also be important to consider the subsidiary stages of reflection, commitment, planning, responsibility, accountability, and then implementation. Exercises, meditation, affirmation, and, above all, practice in differentiating one's choice and becoming aware of compulsive patterns are ways to encourage autonomy and self-directed behaviour in the group.

4   Affirming the idea of service and responsibility in the world counters narcissistic and unhealthy, inward-looking tendencies. Emphasizing the relation of the group experience to the external environment and one's responsibility to others can generate a service ethic which goes beyond members' personal

development. Cultivating a sense of compassion in members for themselves and others is essential, as is the building of an experience of community. I look out for any opportunity which can foster and promote goodwill. The goodwill is a will to do good; it is a will that chooses and wants the good and is thus an expression of love and compassion.

A map for the synthetic groupworker

I think that by now you may have a sense of what I mean when I speak of synthetic groupwork. This is a method and perspective of practice which seeks to activate and engage group members' will and to cultivate the intentional and moral capacity of the individual and the group.

I have said that the worker does this by discriminating between

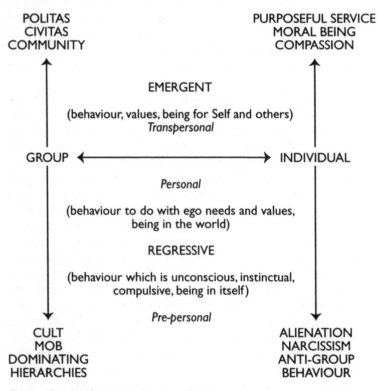

POLITAS
CIVITAS
COMMUNITY

PURPOSEFUL SERVICE
MORAL BEING
COMPASSION

EMERGENT

(behaviour, values, being for Self and others)
Transpersonal

GROUP ←—————————————→ INDIVIDUAL

Personal

(behaviour to do with ego needs and values, being in the world)

REGRESSIVE

(behaviour which is unconscious, instinctual, compulsive, being in itself)

Pre-personal

CULT
MOB
DOMINATING
HIERARCHIES

ALIENATION
NARCISSISM
ANTI-GROUP
BEHAVIOUR

Figure 12.1 A bifocal perspective of group concerns

what is regressive and emergent in group behaviour as a consequence of bringing to bear on phenomena a bifocal vision, which includes a wide range of psychological, psychosocial, existential, and spiritual concerns that many other groupwork models would exclude, reduce, or pathologize. (See figure 12.1.)

This diagram is an attempt to describe and locate individual and group behaviour in terms of whether it is working towards or away from agreed objectives. The vertical axis indicates whether behaviour and intention is regressive or emergent. The horizontal axis indicates the relation and tension between individuals and groups. From this it is possible to look at a phenomenon or incident in the group and ask a range of questions and frame possible interventions:

- Does this event involve an individual and/or the group?
- Is the event regressive or emergent?
- Does it propel the group towards engagement with the political/civic/cultural/spiritual?
- Does the event indicate the presence of cultish, depersonalizing tendencies in the group/sub-grouping and dominating hierarchies?
- Does the event motivate the individual to service, purposeful activity, moral responsibility?
- Does the event indicate individual alienation, narcissistic preoccupation, and anti-group behaviour?

Take some time in your group to ponder and ruminate on these sorts of questions. From such considerations you will be able to decide accurately on what form of intervention best suits the needs and desires of the individuals and the group at any point in time.

Remember that it takes a lot of practice and experience in groups to feel confident with these sorts of questions and interventions, and be prepared to make mistakes and be corrected by the group. This is no disgrace, and can be the basis of the group's learning that it also has responsibility and accountability for its own development and cannot reasonably expect to stay reliant on you.

Review

- Synthetic groupwork encourages a dynamic towards wholeness and emergence.
- Synthetic groupwork emphasizes the expansion of an individual's identity.
- The importance of bifocal vision to differentiate between regressive and emergent psychophysical, psychological, psychosocial, and psychospiritual contexts.

Chapter 13

Keeping your practice going

Putting together all the skills and attitudes that we have been talking about is not an easy business. It takes a great deal of concentration, persistence, and hard work. It means constantly reviewing your practice to see how and where you need to develop next. It means staying in touch with your purpose, refining your vision, and allowing your whole being to be involved in the undertaking. In order to start working with groups and keep your practice going, you must aim to develop a structure which will foster this sort of awareness and generate appropriate strategies for change and learning. Such a structure should rest upon four supporting principles:

- Recording
- Evaluation
- Consultation
- Peer support and training

Let us examine each of these principles and see what is involved.

Recording

Recording is essential and cannot be ignored and yet is an area that seems to present difficulties for both the novice and the more experienced groupworker alike. There appears to be a number of reasons for this.

- Dislike of writing and office work – recording is 'tedious', 'passive', 'boring'
- 'Working' with the group is more exciting
- Recording is synonymous with 'spying', 'surveillance', and 'control'
- The purpose and function of recording is not always clearly thought out and accepted

Whatever the difficulties or objections the importance of recording cannot be stressed sufficiently. Recording serves the following purposes:

- It develops the powers of observation
- It is a means of examining individual and group behaviour and relating this to theoretical knowledge and advice
- It is a means of assessment and evaluation, documenting the growth and development in individuals, groups, and the worker, and providing evidence of action taken and material for future reflection and work
- Recording enables a worker to clarify his thoughts, express feelings and can create deeper awareness and understanding of group situations
- Recording forms a basis for analysing work method, focusing on skills, improving practice, and furthering member involvement and satisfaction
- It is an agency record which indicates the circumstances which precipitated contact, records the work done, over what length of time, and under what conditions, etc.

It is clear then that recording is a tool that can be used to help group members accomplish their goals and to help workers engage in this task. It is not a method of surveillance geared to generate yet more personal information for the authorities nor is it a tiresome chore to get through as quickly as possible. Recording is a way of staying in touch with your vision, developing skills, and learning how to co-operate with members to achieve the purposes for which the group was originally set up.

Guidelines for recording

Useful questions

A lot depends on the purpose of the recording, so ask yourself:

- Who is the recording for – agency, supervisor, colleagues, worker's use, member's use?
- What do these people need to know?
- What is the minimum material to be recorded – individual and group behaviour, performance, interaction; particular incidents; worker interaction, interventions?
- Who will have access to the recordings?

Purpose and objectives

Now make a clear statement about the purpose and objectives of your recording.

Consider who is to record

In some groups, especially when working with children, I find it valuable to involve the group in the recording process. It is a useful way of contextualizing sessions, summarizing work, and teaching skills of process analysis. You can use a rota for recording in the group diary so that each member takes a turn at describing events, or the recording can be made collectively at the end of each session.

Normally, however, this recording does not suit the analysis of worker interventions or group dynamics that you may wish to undertake so a more appropriate record is called for. This record is made by one worker as soon after the session as possible, according to a predetermined format. Where a number of workers co-lead in a group it is important that each worker write a brief personalized account of the session which can be used, or not, to help compile the official history of the session.

I regard records as confidential accounts of the worker's observation and not to be revealed out of context. Members are aware when I record and though I will not show them the recordings, I am prepared to discuss any aspect or detail with them.

Consider the method of recording

In deciding the method that you wish to employ to record it is important to think about:

- The time available to record
- Your ability to recall after the event
- Your ability to summarize
- The availability, relevance, and expertise with technology – video recording, tape recording
- The use to which the recording is to be put

You may feel more comfortable writing up what happened in a session or may prefer to rely on the memory and accuracy of a tape recorder or video camera to capture the essence of the session. If introducing the latter be sure to check out members' fantasies and anxieties about how the material will be used and stored.

I personally prefer the traditional discipline of writing up the session and believe it to be the best method of recording and learning for the novice because in my experience:

- It develops a reflective, critical ability
- Writing stimulates and builds memory retention and recall
- It enables you to mentally rerun the group, clarifies thinking, and develops understanding of process and interaction
- It is a marvellous method of self-evaluation and training in the absence of a suitable supervisor
- Writing builds discipline, rigour, and concentration
- It helps formulate future objectives and strategies
- It provides opportunity for expression of feeling, resolution, and the emergence of meaning

Recording what goes on in groups

There are many ways of recording and analysing what people do in groups. You can use sociograms, analyse interaction according to certain categories, observe the task- and group-oriented behaviours of members (see Chapter 3, page 71), and the like. The following framework can be used as a general guide to recording with your group:

- *Basic identifying information*: State name of group, date, time of session, those present, absent.
- *State session objectives*: Your desired outcomes and what you hope to accomplish in the session.
- *State the session programme and methodology you intend to use.*
- *Content analysis of session*: This is a straightforward narrative account of what occurred in the session. This gives a context for exploring process or particular incidents and interventions later on.
- *Process analysis of session*: This section allows for consideration and reflection of group dynamics. It is a qualitative analysis of what was happening. It can focus on:

- Process analysis of individual and group interaction in the session
- A particular event or the major incidents
- Themes such as communication, participation, relationships, power and influence, trust
- A set of actions or interventions undertaken by workers

The section on working with process on page 189, Chapter 8, will give you headings and advice on what to write and how to organize this portion of the record.

The following headings are also useful as a framework for recording:

- *Individual commentaries*: Include a brief description of each member's progress in that session. Consider their investment in the group, behaviour, performance, attitudes, and relationships. How are they working towards their personal goals and what help do they need?
- *Workers' intervention*: Consider the contribution and interventions of workers in the group. What was good, valuable, what was ill-timed, irrelevant, or off the mark? What skills do you need to develop or train up? How did you get on with

co-workers? What was good about this? What was avoided? What needs to be reviewed?

- *Evaluative comment on session*: This is a general résumé of what took place, perhaps locating the session in some developmental context or stages theory. Indicate whether session objectives were achieved, what remains to be done, or needs to be renegotiated. How did programme work? What needs to be reviewed? What are your future objectives, plans?

By recording in this way you will have a full and comprehensive picture of what is happening in your group and can assess how your practice is hindering or facilitating this. In the absence of a supervisor or peer support, recording is an invaluable tool and may well be the only method available for training, so do begin now to pay more attention to the contribution that recording can make to keeping your practice going.

Evaluation

There are two aspects of evaluation which are of direct relevance to your ability to keep your practice going. The first concerns the way in which you evaluate change or progress within the group and this is group- or member-oriented. The second has to do with how you evaluate your own practice and performance and is worker-oriented. Let us look at this more closely.

Evaluating the group

The idea dies hard that evaluation is something that you only do at the end of the group. In Chapter 2 I suggested that evaluation has to be considered during the planning phase and before the group has been set up (see page 43).

Evaluation is a way of assessing:

- Outcomes – the extent to which the group has achieved its goals in producing change/learning, etc.
- Service delivery – the relevance, quality, acceptability of group work in a particular setting
- Structure and process of the group – what actually happened in the group, how it was organized, how resources were used, and the like

Do not allow yourself to be put off by the thought of evaluating the group experience. It need not be complicated. The basic requirements for an evaluation study are:

> • The establishment of a baseline from which the programme starts
> • A record of the input of effort
> • An account of any movement from the baseline
> • Follow-up to see if change has been maintained

Within these principles you have a great deal of latitude in terms of how you go about assessing the group contribution. Even if not required to by your agency, it is worthwhile evaluating because it will provide you with thoughtful and rich insights into the nature and power of groups and will give you plenty of material to think about in terms of your own practice.

Here are some things to think about when considering how to evaluate the group.

What kind of information is needed?

The only rationale for collecting information is to answer specific questions which have been thought out well in advance. Inevitably a lot more information will be collected in the course of normal recording than will be used so it is worthwhile composing definite questions at the start or working to a framework through which information can be filtered. (See section on recording in this chapter.)

Ask yourself: what is it specifically that I want to know about individual or group?

> • Behaviour
> • Skills
> • Attitudes
> • Values
> • Feelings
> • Goals

Make a list of questions that you can work with.

Consider if particular questions, frameworks, or measurements are:

- Appropriate
- Reliable
- Valid
- Easy to use and understand

It should be clear by now that the first step in the evaluation process is the early and explicit identification of the outcomes that the group is being set up to produce. These outcomes can refer to goal attainment, improved functioning, or effectiveness and to certain specified changes in the targets of intervention. Outcomes should be defined operationally and should state as correctly as possible:

- Just how you could tell if a person had developed more self-awareness and insight
  or
- What a person would do who had acquired new social skills
  or
- How you would know if members had benefited from group support and caring

Consider who will be your sources of information

You can collect information from:

- Group members
- Worker observations
- Co-workers
- Significant others – parents, teachers, peers, colleagues, etc.

Consider how the information is to be obtained

There is a great diversity and range of methods for data collection. Amongst other methods, you can use:

- Direct observation of behaviour
- Surveys and questionnaires
- Personality tests and self-rating scales
- Formal or informal interviews
- Analysis of records, documents, and projects
- Sociometric devices

The important thing to remember here is that the instruments used must actually measure what you want them to, so do link the instruments specifically to your questions.

When will the information be obtained and recorded?

The purpose of evaluation will help you decide the timing and sequence of data collection. If you are measuring outcomes you will need a baseline at the start of the group which can be contrasted with information gathered at the end of the group. Evaluating the process of the group will require much more frequent and periodic assessment.

It is usually best to record information as close to the event as possible so anticipate that you will require a recording period after sessions and allow sufficient time.

Consider how you intend to use the information

You need to summarize the information collected and draw conclusions, create meaning, make statements, comparisons, and predictions and show if the work has value or not. Generally I use the information to:

- Abstract generalizations and relationships
- Generate working principles
- Adjust programme, goals, methodology
- Provide feedback and comparison for members, agency, significant others
- Provide learning, training, skill development
- Determine success, relevance, etc., of group

You can use collected information at the end of the group to make a thorough and final evaluation of the experience. It is also worth considering the building in of review periods every six to eight sessions in order to:

- See if plans are being carried out
- Determine if objectives are being met
- Reassess needs
- Realign to purpose
- Set fresh or more realistic objectives and plans

This can become a cyclical process which contributes to group functioning, and can if the reviews are recorded, generate much valuable material for comparison and analysis later.

Involve members

Consider ways of encouraging the active participation of members where possible in the evaluative process. Any evaluation is time-consuming and depends on its respondents for its richness and relevance, so involving members is a good way of sharing the load and enriching the results. You may have to negotiate issues about confidentiality with group members and set boundaries on how the information being collected will be used and presented so as to preserve anonymity and the like. Make appropriate contracts and agreements which will reassure people and engage them in a process of ongoing assessment and realignment.

Encourage members to keep a personal journal where they can record, draw, or describe significant events, experiences, and insights in the group. These contemporaneous records can be augmented by the group diary records of project work, and periodic reviews to help determine whether change or improvement occurred during the life of the group. They also create a climate in which people experience evaluation as an integral part of group membership and see it contributing to group well-being and improved functioning.

Evaluating and teaching yourself

Once you begin to work with a group you can both evaluate yourself and get feedback from members and others on how you are doing. In this way you can begin to initiate a programme of self-training which will enable you to keep your practice fresh, innovative, and relevant.

The important thing to remember, however, is that you have to work at it – hard! Your practice will develop in an orderly and comprehensible manner only if you take responsibility for it and that means approaching your handling of groups in a thoughtful and organized way. Here are some guidelines which will help you evaluate and change your practice.

Keep a journal

Keep a personal journal in which you can jot down your thoughts, feelings, experiences, and insights in the group. Reread it constantly. Gradually you will find certain themes recurring. It may be something that you become aware you are avoiding or mishandling. It could be a situation which makes you anxious or uncomfortable.

Choose one problem area that you wish to work on

Without altering or changing in any way, begin to be more conscious of how this behaviour, attitude, or feeling manifests in the group. Gather information about this problem area. Try to identify stages, elements, or parts in the process. Can you recognize the imminence of the behaviour or feeling? What happens as the situation develops? What is it like for you afterwards? If it is appropriate, invite feedback from members or others on how they see you in a particular situation:

> I'm wondering if I come in too quickly sometimes to help you sort things out. What do you think about this?

Subsequent feedback will create a bigger, more detailed, and specific picture of what you are doing and may suggest options and possibilities.

You can also obtain feedback by asking members to fill in reaction forms or short questionnaires about specific topics at the end of sessions. Best of all is to cultivate an environment in which members feel it is permissible and even a friendly act to comment in a mature way about aspects of your practice.

Create a vision

Ask yourself why you want to develop your skill or ability in a particular area.

- Why do you need to change?
- What is the problem?
- Why is it a problem?
- Why is it a problem now?

Your answers to these questions serve two valuable functions:

- They tell you what, specifically, you are dissatisfied with and why this is so. Knowing what you want to develop or change begins to open up possibilities and can create a vision or sense of how you might behave differently. And as we have seen in Chapter 8, page 159, vision creates goals.
- Goals are always important and never more so than when you are trying to maintain yourself in your practice. Goals motivate because they promise rewards. Only the promise of behaving or intervening in a more effective way is going to get you to put in the necessary work to alter or modify an existing behaviour. So spend some time motivating yourself and determining why it is worthwhile to change.

Make your vision concrete

Rather than trying to change a number of things in your practice, work on one area at a time. To do this, sit down with pen and paper and write down a statement of the problem, your goal, or vision. Do a short brainstorming session and write down whatever ideas come to your mind as good possibilities. Do not think too hard about it. Just let the ideas come. Now take another sheet of paper and write at the top, 'My ideal model'. Write a paragraph or two describing an ideal image of yourself behaving or acting in a particular way.

I often find it useful at this stage to use some of the visualization techniques discussed in Chapter 10, page 215. A few minutes imagining or visualizing myself performing in a certain way gives the feel of the behaviour, affirms its value, and engages the will to change in the desired direction.

Now read over what you have written, then take a fresh sheet of paper. Based on what seems most meaningful from the ideal scene you have created above, make a list of three or four important goals in the problem area. You can then prioritize these goals in terms of what is most urgent, easiest, or worthy of attention. Choose one aspect and resolve to start with it.

Planning the change

The next thing to do is to acknowledge any feelings you may have about your specific goal which could hinder your progress. Feelings of fear, inadequacy, shame, and the like can create impotence and despair if not dealt with. An important way of handling such feelings is to reconnect to your original vision and draw strength from it. This affirms the value and rightness of your course.

It can also be useful to make a list of the things that will prevent you reaching your goal as it may well be that there are certain factors or a particular sequence of actions that must be considered before you start to initiate change.

Be sure to compile an equal list of things that will help you move forwards to your goal so that you can utilize and build on your positive abilities. It is worth reviewing the section on problem solving in Chapter 5, page 115 and in particular the discussion of 'force-field analysis' as there are some ideas which will help you plan a change programme.

From your programme determine your next realistic step and then initiate your change strategies one move at a time.

Evaluate progress

Because you have been specific at the goal-setting stage you can, after a predetermined period, assess how you have been getting on with altering or modifying your practice. If you find that you have not made as much progress as you thought, which will sometimes happen, do not get disheartened or assume that you have failed. Acknowledge to yourself that you still have not achieved your goal and consider whether it really is something that you want. You may have to repeat several of the above steps (choosing a problem area, creating a vision, and making it concrete) to determine whether you want to set the goal again or let it go.

It is important to acknowledge and work with unaccomplished goals in this way. Otherwise they will accumulate and leave you with a sense of inadequacy and failure which will eventually result in you avoiding evaluation and change in your practice. The key is always to choose only those goals that you genuinely want and will give you satisfaction.

When you find that you have achieved a goal, even it is small, be sure to acknowledge this and find a way of rewarding yourself. Rewards are what will motivate you and give you the strength and desire to continue developing your practice.

The process which I have outlined is an invaluable and essential part of your professional practice with groups and – particularly in the absence of supervision or training – will help you.

- See evaluation as an integral part of your work
- Obtain practice in goal setting and the management of change
- Get in touch with and clarify the important purposes and direction in your practice

---

Do try to develop the habit of constantly evaluating and monitoring your own practice. You will find that it pays very rich dividends.

Consultation

You must assume responsibility for your own professional growth and evolution. No one can develop your practice for you. You must do the work yourself. But at times it can be a painful and difficult experience and you will need support, guidance, and encouragement. So assuming responsibility for your professional growth involves setting up a support system which will contain you while you question and examine your practice. This is where the consultant comes in.

I use the word consultant instead of supervisor because I want to stress the importance of your personal choice and volition in keeping your practice going. The supervisor is one who is primarily obliged to hold you to account for your work, although he may help you unfold your practice. While being accountable for one's work is essential it is more your responsibility for developing and promoting practice that I want to emphasize here. So the idea of consultant as one who is sought out as opposed to the supervisor who seeks out the practitioner, is more appropriate.

In order to keep your practice going and growing it is important that you engage with a more experienced worker who is prepared to help you look critically at what you do in groups. Ideally such a worker will have worked with groups and will be aware of the process and dynamics of collective behaviour. This worker will know from his own experience what is likely to happen at certain times in the group, may have some helpful ideas about current and apparently incomprehensible events, and will usually be able to guide you through the sandbars, shallows, and rapids of groupwork.

Often, however, it may not be possible to find someone in your agency experienced enough or willing to act as a consultant for you.

In these circumstances look around for a worker that you admire – someone who attracts you by virtue of his excellence or competence in his own field. A person like this can still help you a great deal even if he has not worked in groups. His experience and ability in his own sphere of activity will enable him to ask penetrating and stimulating questions which will give you a novel and fresh perspective on your practice.

Your practice consultant should be able to provide you with a safe, stimulating, and supportive environment in which you can:

- Consider an alternative, rational, and objective viewpoint on your practice
- Analyse the process and dynamics of group membership
- Consider and align with your purpose or vision
- Work from the known to the unknown, from the apparent to the hidden
- Learn to recognize inappropriate reactions and behaviours
- Explore your inner conflicts
- Experience your hidden feelings
- Experiment with new behaviour and attitudes
- Plan and execute strategies
- Find refreshment, strength, and nourishment

Using consultation

Before the session

Prepare yourself and your consultant by writing up the group session that you want to look at or forwarding any appropriate notes, tapes, or video recordings. It is useful to review your practice and identify any concerns or areas of work that you want to examine. Make an agenda for yourself. Sometimes in consultation you may find that there are issues or feelings that you avoid discussing or which emerge after your session. It is important to bring this unfinished business with you to the next session as your consultant cannot read your mind and this material can get in the way. It is up to you to keep the lines of communication open and clear.

During the session

Agree with the consultant an agenda of mutual concerns about your practice that can be discussed in the session. Clear any unfinished business. Be alert for any tendency on your part to impress, over-react, or try to change your consultant. If you are doing this with him you are probably doing this in your group or experiencing this with members and it is important to explore the motivations and feelings behind this behaviour. Some of the more common patterns that I have seen in my role as consultant are:

- Demand that the consultant give a prescription, magic formula, or answer endless questions
- Avoid, neglect, or ignore the consultant's suggestions
- Pretend to accept the consultant's suggestions when they seem incorrect or incomprehensible
- Fantasy that he can read your mind
- Blame him because he cannot understand you
- Keep the discussion at a safe or superficial level

Very often I have seen workers bring to the consultation and act out the behaviours and resistances that they themselves manifest or experience with members in the group. For this reason, it is wise to be alert to your feelings about the consultant since how you manage them between you, will offer valuable insight and suggestion for handling similar feelings and behaviours in your group.

After the session

The consultant will stir up emotions, stimulate, and provide you with a wealth of material and advice. Plan to take some quiet time afterwards where you can sit and write in your journal. Make notes under headings such as:

- What I am doing well
- What I am weak in
- What I missed/avoided in the group
- What I am going to watch for/work with in the next group session
- Goals: short, medium, long-range
- How I felt about consultation/consultant
- Unfinished business
- What I appreciate about myself in consultation/last group session

---

The point is to give some time to planning how, and what you are going to do about what came up in the consultation because if it is to be meaningful, you have to act on what you learned in these sessions. Genuine change in your practice comes about from the combination of insight plus new behaviour so do take time to consider specifically how you intend to use what is emerging in consultation.

In deciding to work with groups then resolve to build in a consultative dimension for your practice. But remember, consultation is an aid and support to your practice. It is not a substitute for hard work. It will enhance but not replace your responsibility for keeping your practice going.

Peer support and training

Another source of support, guidance, and encouragement for your practice is your colleagues and fellow workers. It is really important that you acquaint people in your work setting of your intention to run a group in order to secure their co-operation and ensure that you have the time and resource to work. As the group meets and starts to unfold, keep your colleagues informed of what is going on. Consider giving occasional verbal reports at a staff meeting, informal discussion of how you experience working with a group, short written reports, and the like. In this way you will involve other colleagues and interest them in your work. You will find then that in times of crisis or difficulty you have a sympathetic and knowledge-able support group to fall back on. Be careful, however, not to bore other people or flood the market with accounts of your work!

Outside your immediate work setting look for other group workers or people who are interested in working with groups. Get to know them, ask for advice with problems, and talk to them about their philosophy, technique, and style. Exchange views, books, tips, and begin to develop an informal network of support and resource. Try to set up a peer support group if possible. Even if there are only three or four members, such a group can be a valuable means of challenging yourself, puzzling out problems in your practice, and developing a sense of community. This sense or feeling of belonging to a groupwork community is very important. Very often novice group workers can feel isolated or separate from their colleagues by virtue of their interest in groups. In addition the characteristics and peculiarities of groupwork practice can also heighten the sense of separateness or difference. So contact and exchange with other group workers is a way of preserving and maintaining your practice particularly in adverse or hostile conditions. It is also worthwhile joining local or national groupwork associations which not only offer support, but also provide opportunities for further training.

These associations often offer short training courses which will help you develop your skills, reflect on your practice, and make new contacts. A word of advice: do not 'collect' two or three training courses in the hope of suddenly acquiring instant skills. Do one course and then aim to give yourself six months to a year to decide that in the next two groups you will experiment with and try out what you have been taught. In this way each training course that you do deepens and expands your practice in a mature and system-atic manner.

Consider joining an experiential group which will give you the opportunity to feel what it is like to be a member amongst others in the group. This will provide rich insights and perceptions into interpersonal dynamics that will serve you well in your own practice. Join groups where you know good leaders are to be found. Study closely the style and technique of as many group leaders across as broad a spectrum as you can. Ask yourself continually:

- Why did he do/say that?
- What would I have said/done in that situation?
- What makes this leader good?
- What do I like about him?
- What do I not like about him?
- What can I borrow/adopt/modify from his style?

You do not have to give up your own individuality or become a clone of a certain group leader in order to adapt from his style. Give yourself permission to borrow parts of other people's way of working and then piece them together in your own unique style.

Look constantly for ways of being in contact with other people doing groupwork and learn from them. In this way you can minimize and cushion yourself from the inevitable hurts and challenges of working with a group of people while at the same time, ensuring that your practice is innovative, vital, and alive.

Survival procedures for creative group workers

Rule 1: Avoid crucifixions

This rule counsels against over-involvement or self-sacrifice in any cause which you do not wish to be your last. You are not a messiah nor are group members your disciples. So do not try to save, protect, rescue, or work it out for everyone all of the time. It is difficult to watch another person in pain or see them make what appears to be an avoidable error but often this is an essential part of their growth and you can best help by allowing it to happen. Avoid being seen as a saviour, guru, or charismatic leader because we crucify our messiahs, shoot our presidents, and forget our pop stars more quickly than you would find comfortable.

Rule 2: Don't push the river upstream

The essence of this rule is that you should learn to avoid working in any way which will energize resistance to the course or path that you believe is desirable. There seems to be a law of inverse effort which applies when you work in groups. People seem to be contrary. The more you do the less they do; the more helpful you try to be, the more they cling to their unhelpful beliefs. What is required is a light and sensitive touch because it is insistence, short-sightedness, and dogmatism on your part which will generate resistance amongst group members. So do not force encounters or tell people what to do. Learn to work from where the group is at. Go with the flow.

Rule 3: Wait quietly until the mud settles

Learn to wait and watch and listen. In this way your awareness is focused on the group and not just on your needs. Do not feel you should intervene immediately – stand back until you know what is happening in a situation. Keep quiet, remain attentive, and take things as they come. When you know what people want – or are repulsed by – then you can move and show them how they can get what they want by doing what you want them to do.

Rule 4: Learn to forgive yourself

In the course of working with groups it is inevitable that you will make mistakes and feel inadequate at times. Feelings of helplessness and confusion, shame, anger, and pain will frequently arise and threaten to overwhelm unless you can cultivate a sense of right proportion and be compassionate with yourself.

Be respectful of yourself as someone who is learning a difficult and demanding craft. Begin to see and use mistakes as a source of creativity and an opportunity to learn new skills and try out new behaviours. Learn to forgive yourself since if you cannot permit your own frailty and inadequacy you will really be unable to allow it in your group. Learn how to connect to the power of your own helplessness!

Rule 5: Cultivate goodwill

Keep in awareness why you thought the group was a good idea originally and use this vision to express goodwill towards group members. At various times members will attempt to please, shock, manipulate, and help you. There is no point in getting angry or hurt at this and rejecting them. This will only compound matters. Learn to accept members and help them explore these self-defeating behaviours and discover more positive and creative ways of being. Your job is to guide and facilitate the group, not join members in destructive relationships. So act with optimism and goodwill and teach by example.

Rule 6: Make up your own rules

No book or course can give you the complete prescription for working with a group. Every group is different, though there are similar patterns and themes. You will find yourself in situations which are not covered in this work and are new to you. Do not be afraid to improvise, break the normal rules, or go against the conventional wisdom. Use your imagination and intuition to guess at what is the best thing to do. If it doesn't work fall back on rules one, three, and four. If it does work incorporate it into your repertoire and forget about it! The important thing to remember is that you do the best you can and let it go at that. Rule 6 could have been rewritten as 'there are no rules'. It is your group so adapt, modify, create in your own fashion. If it works, use it! If it fails to work, use that too!

The last word

Writing this book has been for me analogous to working with a group. I entered the work full of vision, hope, and optimism. After a time the going became very tough and it was tempting to give up. But I persevered and as you see the work is complete. As always the difficulties arose from my attempts to make the work go where I wanted it to go. It is only to the degree that I have succeeded in letting go of my needs to impress, control, and expound that I have learned to co-operate with the process of the writing. Just like working with a group. May you learn the same lesson.

Notes and references

Introduction

1 Hargreaves, D.H. (1972) *Interpersonal Relations and Education (PH)*, London: Routledge & Kegan Paul.
2 Davies, B. (1975) *The Use of Groups in Social Work Practice*. 58, London: Routledge & Kegan Paul.
3 For a review of definitions of groups see Cartwright, D. and Zander, A. (eds) (1968) *Group Dynamics, Research, and Theory*, London: Tavistock.
4 Ferrucci, P. (1982) *What we may be*, England: Turnstone Press. Whitmore, D. (1986) *Psychosynthesis in Education*, England: Turnstone Press.
Assagioli, R. (1975) *Psychosynthesis*, England: Turnstone Press.

I How to plan the group

1 Whitaker, D.S (1976) 'Some conditions for effective work in groups', *British Journal of Social Work*, 5, 4: 249.
2 Douglas, T. (1976) *Groupwork Practice*: 41, London: Tavistock Publications.
3 Douglas, T. (1976) op. cit., p. 41.
4 Lowy, L. (1972) 'Goal formulation in social work with groups', in Bernstein (ed.) *Further Explorations in Group Work*: 128, London: Bookstall.
5 Whitaker, D.S. (1976) op. cit., p. 426.
6 Parsloe, P. (1971) 'What social workers say in groups of clients', *British Journal of Social Work*, 1, 1: 39.
7 Whitaker, D.S. (1976) op. cit., p. 423.
8 Paradise, R. and Daniels, R. (1972) 'Group composition as a treatment tool with children', in S. Bernstein (ed.) *Further Explorations in Groupwork*, London: Bookstall.
9 Bertcher, H.J. and Maple, F. (1974) 'Elements and issues in group composition', in P. Glasser, R. Sarri, and R. Vinter, *Individual Change Through Small Groups*, New York: Free Press.
10 Tropp, E. (1976) 'A developmental theory', in R. Roberts and

H. Northen (eds) *Theories for Social Work with Groups*: 217, New York: Columbia University Press.

11 Ibid., p. 217.
12 Ibid., p. 217.
13 McCullough, M.K. and Ely, P.J. (1971) *Social Work with Groups*: 6, London: Routledge & Kegan Paul.
14 Berelson, B. and Steiner, G.A. (1964) *Human Behaviour: An Inventory of Scientific Findings*: 360, New York: Harcourt.
15 Parad, H.J., Selby, L., and Quinlan, J. (1976) 'Crisis intervention with families and groups', in R. Roberts, and H. Northen (eds), op. cit.
16 Vinter, R.D. (1974) 'Program activities: an analysis of their effects on participant behaviour', *Individual Change through Small Groups*, op. cit., p. 233.
17 Ross, A.L. and Bernstein, N.D. (1976) 'A framework for the therapeutic use of group activities', *Child Welfare*, LV, 9: 627–39.
18 Vinter, R.D. (1974) op. cit.

2 Leading and setting up the group

1 For more detailed discussion on styles of leadership see Hartford, N.E. (1976) 'Group methods and generic practice', in R.W. Roberts and H. Northen (eds) *Theorics for Social Work with Groups*, New York: Columbia University Press.
2 For a detailed account of evaluation approaches and techniques see Thomas, J. *et al.* (1981) 'Goal-setting and evaluation', in M.R. Whitlam (ed.) *Practice Development Papers*, National Intermediate Treatment Federation.
3 Hodge, J. (1977) 'Social groupwork: rules for establishing the group', *Social Work Today*, 8, 17: 110.
4 Schwarz, W. (1976) 'Between client and system: the mediating approach', in *Theories for Social Work with Groups*, op. cit.

3 An introduction to group dynamics and process

1 Lerner, I. (1976) *Diary of the Way: Three Paths to Enlightenment*: 26, New York: Ridge Press.
2 Maslow, A. (1954) *Motivation and Personality*, New York: Harper & Row.
3 Berne, K.D. and Sheats, P. (1948) 'Functional roles of group members', *Journal of Social Issues*, 4, 2: 41–9.
4 Underwood, W. (1970) 'Roles that facilitate and inhibit group development', in R.T. Golembiewski, and A. Blumberg (eds) *Sensitivity Training and The Laboratory Approach: Readings about Concepts and Applications*, Itasca IL: Peacock.
5 Bogdanoff, M. and Elbaum, O.L. (1978) 'Role lock . . . monopolisers, mistrusters, isolates, Helpful Hannahs, and other assorted characters in group psychotherapy', *International Journal of Group Psychotherapy*, 28, 2: 247–62.
6 Sarri, R.C. and Galinsky, M.J. (1974) 'A conceptual framework for

group development', in P. Glasser, R.C. Sarri, and R. Vinter, *Individual Change Through Small Groups*: 71–86, New York: Free Press.

7 Assagioli, R. (1983) *Psychosynthesis Typology: Psychosynthesis Monograph*: 27, London: Institute of Psychosynthesis.

8 Angyal, A. (1969) *Foundations for a Science of Personality*: 172, New York: Viking Compass.

9 Ibid.

10 Assagioli, R. (1983) op. cit., p. 21.

11 Schutz, W. (1979) *Profound Simplicity*: 111–37, London: Turnstone Books.

12 Tuckman, B.W. (1965) 'Developmental sequence in small groups', *Psychological Bulletin*, 63, 6: 384–99.

13 Garland, J., Jones, H., and Kolodny, K. (1965) 'A model for stages in the development of social work groups', in S. Bernstein (ed.) *Explorations in Group Work*, London: Bookstall.

14 Ibid., p. 35.

15 Ibid., p. 43.

16 Hartford, M.E. (1972) 'Phases in group development', *Groups in Social Work: Application of Small Group Theory and Research to Social Work Practice*: 63–93, New York: Columbia University Press.

17 Blofeld, J. (1968) *I Ching: The Chinese Book of Changes*: 185, London: Allen & Unwin.

18 Ibid., p. 201.

19 Tuckman, B.W. op. cit., p. 396.

20 Ibid., p.396.

8 The foundations of creative groupwork

1 Butler, T. and Fuhriman, A. (1983) 'Curative factors in group therapy: a review of the recent literature', *Small Group Behaviour*, 14 2: 131–42.

2 Yalom, I.D. (1970) *The Theory and Practice of Group Psychotherapy*, New York: Basic Books.

3 Frankl, V. (1963) *Man's search for meaning*, New York: Pocket Books.

4 Klein, A.T. (1972) *Effective Groupwork*, New York: Association Press.

5 Assagioli, R. (1980) *Psychosynthesis: A Collection of Basic Writings*: 131, Wellingborough: Turnstone Books.

10 The techniques of creative groupwork

1 Quoted in Baynes, C.F. (1950) trans., *The I Ching or Book of Changes*, Princeton, New Jersey: Princeton University Press.

2 • Badaines, J. (1977) 'Psychodrama: acting your problems away', *Psychology Today*, December: 38–40.

• Badaines, J. (1977) 'Psychodrama: concepts, principles, and issues, *Drama Therapy*, 1, 2.

• Keysell, P. (1975) *Motives for Mime*, London: Evans.

• Pemberton-Billing, R.N. and Clegs, J.D. (1968) *Teaching Drama*, London: University of London Press.

- Rayner, P. (1976) 'Psychodrama as a medium for intermediate treatment', *British Journal of Social Work*, 7, 4: 443–53.
- Way, B. (1975) *Development Through Drama*, London: Longman.

3
- Goodnow, J. (1977) *Children's Drawing*, London: Fontana.
- Liebman, M. (1982) *Art Games and Structures for Groups*, Bristol: Bristol Art Therapy Group.
- Oaklander, V. (1978) *Windows to Our Children*, esp. pp. 21–52, Moab, Utah: Real People Press.
- Remocker, J. and Storch, E. (1979) *Action Speaks Louder*, Edinburgh: Churchill Livingstone.
- Storr; A. (1976) *The Dynamics of Creation*, Harmondsworth: Pelican.

4 Assagioli, R. (1980) *Psychosynthesis*, esp. Chapter 5, London: Wildwood House.

5 Assagioli, R. (1980) *The Act of Will*, esp. Chapter 5, London: Wildwood House.

6 Ferrucci, P. (1982) *The Visions and Techniques of Psychosynthesis*, Wellingborough: Turnstone Press.

7 op. cit., p. 144 ff.

8 op. cit., p. 167 ff.

9 Whitmore, D. (1986) *Psychosynthesis in Education*, Wellingborough: Turnstone Press.

10 Fugitt, E.D. (1983) *He Hit Me Back First: Creative Visualization Activities for Parenting and Teaching*, California: Jalmar Press.

11 De Mille, R. (1972) *Put Your Mother on the Ceiling*, New York: Viking Press.

12 Gawain, S. (1978) *Creative Visualization*, Millvalley, CA: Whatever Publishing.

13 Masters, R.E.L. and Houston, J. (1983) *Mindgames: The Guide to Inner Space*, Wellingborough: Dover Publications.

14 See:

- Brandes, D. and Phillips, H. (1979), *Gamester's Handbook*, London: Hutchinson.
- De Boro, E. (1980) *Lateral Thinking*, Harmondsworth: Penguin.
- Hopson, B. and Hough, P. (C.R.A.C., 1973) *Exercises in Personal and Career Development*, Cambridge: Hobsons Press.
- Jelfs, M. *Manual for Action*, 128 Bethnal Green Road, London: Action Resources Group.
- Pfeiffer, J.W. and Jones, J.E. (1975) *Handbook of Structured Experiences for Human Relations Training*, 5 vols, USA: University Associates, Publishers, and Consultants.
- Stevens, J.O. (1973) *Awareness*, USA: Bantam Books.

15 For an introduction to sculpting read:

Hopkins, J. (1981) 'Seeing yourself as others see you', *Social Work Today*, 12, 25:10–13.

16 For more on poetry and creative writing, see:

Carradice, P. (1981) 'Ode to a tiger', *Social Work Today*, 13, 7: 22–3.

For journalling techniques, see:

- Progoff, I. (1978) *At a Journal Workshop*, New York: Dialogue House Library.
- Rainwater, J. (1979) *You're in Charge*, Chapter 4, Wellingborough: Turnstone Press.

II Working more intensively with groups

1 Sandler, J., Dare. C., and Holder, A. (1979) *The Patient and the Analyst*, chap. 4, 'Transference' London: Maresfield Reprints.
2 Rycroft, C. (1983) *A Critical Dictionary of Psychoanalysis*, London: Penguin, p. 125.
3 Storr, A., (1975) *Jung*, chap. 3, 'Archetypes and the Collective Unconscious', Collins: Fontana Modern Masters.
4 Foulkes, S.H., (1984) *Therapeutic Group Analysis*, London: Maresfield Reprints, p. 292.
5 Foulkes, S.H. (1984) op. cit., p. 290.
6 Sandler, J. *et al.* (1979) op. cit., chap. 6, 'Counter-transference'.

12 Working more synthetically with the group

1 Assagioli, R. (1980) *Psychosynthesis: A Collection of Basic Writings*, Wellingborough: Turnstone Press.
2 Assagioli, R. (1980) *The Act of Will*, London: Wildwood House.
3 Fukuyama, M.A. and Sevig, T.D. (1999) *Integrating Spirituality into Multicultural Counselling*, London: Sage Publications, p. 9.
4 Yalom, I.D. (1980) *Existential Psychotherapy*, New York: Basic Books.
5 Fromm, E. (1960) *Fear of Freedom*, London: Routledge & Kegan Paul.
6 Frankl, V. (1963) *Man's Search for Meaning*, New York: Pocket Books.

Name index

Subject index